Textbook of Veterinary Homeopathy

John Saxton
BVetMed, VetFFHom, CertIAVH, MRCVS

Peter Gregory
BVSc, VetFFHom, CertIAVH, MRCVS

BEACONSFIELD PUBLISHERS LTD
Beaconsfield, Bucks, UK

First published in 2005

Email: books@beaconsfield-publishers.co.uk
Website: www.beaconsfield-publishers.co.uk

British Library Cataloguing in Publication Data
Saxton, John
    Textbook of veterinary homeopathy. – (The Beaconsfield
        homeopathic library; no. 24)
    1. Homeopathic veterinary medicine
    I. Title   II. Gregory, Peter
    636´.0895532

    ISBN 0–906584–57–4

Typeset by Gem Graphics, Trenance, Cornwall in 10 on 12¼ point Times
Printed and bound in Great Britain at The Alden Press, Oxford

Acknowledgements

To my wife, Pat, for her constant encouragement, forbearance and much useful advice.   J.S.

To my father, for teaching me more than I realised, and to Cher who showed me the Way and shared the journey.   P.G.

The authors also wish to thank their colleagues Christopher Day, Douglas Wilson, Francis Hunter, Kirsten Brock and Susan Wynn for reading a late draft of the manuscript and offering many helpful comments, and our fellow partners at the Homeopathic Professionals Teaching Group for their support and friendship. Our thanks too to Dr Peter Fisher, editor of the *British Homoeopathic Journal* (now *Homeopathy*) for his kind permission to quote from several issues. Finally, to John Churchill of Beaconsfield Publishers, for his help and patience in guiding two virgin authors through to a successful parturition.

Preface

This book grew out of the Homeopathic Professionals Teaching Group, as two of the veterinary tutors connected with the course realised that there is no current work that is directed at veterinary surgeons, whereas there are texts available which aim to cater for the needs of doctors. Such veterinary works as do exist are directed mainly at animal owners. Whilst these have a certain value for veterinary surgeons, they fall short of what is needed by the committed student. This book attempts to fulfil the needs of the increasing number of veterinary surgeons with a genuine interest in homeopathy, providing sufficient information for them to gain an understanding of the principles and philosophy, together with guidance on basic prescribing. At the same time it is hoped that both the more experienced veterinary practitioner and colleagues in other medical professions will find useful information in it.

It is assumed that the reader has no previous knowledge of homeopathy. Inevitably some information, especially that pertaining to basic principles, will be available in other texts. However, as one of the aims has been to draw together material that is otherwise scattered throughout the literature, homeopaths of all disciplines should find it of value. Emphasis is given to the veterinary aspects of all subjects. Thus different routes to the simillimum which are particularly useful in animals are discussed to a greater degree than in the purely human texts. The emphasis throughout is on basic principles that can be applied to all situations. Detailed discussion of individual species, especially the farm animals, is only included where the approach differs from the standard.

In the main, detailed materia medica has been omitted. This aspect of homeopathy is well covered in other works, and its principal mention here is within the context of the veterinary dimension. The aim has been to provide an introductory manual and reference work that will not sit unthumbed on shelves for too long, but which will be well used, encouraging and informing the aspiring veterinary homeopath and assisting in the creation of a rounded practitioner capable of operating at all levels of homeopathic prescribing.

Contents

PART I: THE THEORY

Chapter 1

The History of Homeopathy

What is Homeopathy?

Homeopathy is a system of medicine, the philosophy of which differs considerably from that of orthodox medicine. This does not mean that the two are always incompatible; indeed there are occasions where they may even work in synergy, but homeopathy does offer a very different way of understanding the process of disease and its treatment by medical means. Homeopathic medicine can be of value across the whole spectrum of disease in animals, either used alone or as a complementary therapy to other forms of treatment, and is indeed capable of resolving conditions which would otherwise be considered incurable, or at the very least intractable. As an introduction to the concepts involved in homeopathy it may be helpful to consider it from a historical perspective.

So firstly let us define what we mean by 'homeopathy'. The word is derived from the Greek words 'homoios' and 'pathos' meaning 'similar' and 'suffering' respectively; the principle of homeopathy therefore is that disease in an organism may be cured by the administration of a substance which, when given to a healthy individual, would induce similar symptoms.

In contrast, much of orthodox medicine is 'antipathic' (where the effects of the medicine are contrary to the symptoms) or 'allopathic' (where the effect of the medicine bears no relationship to the symptoms). For instance, the treatment of diarrhoea with a constipating agent

---

Footnote. The classical spelling of the word includes the diphthong 'œ' (thus 'homœopathy'), or the simpler form 'oe' ('homoeopathy'). American spelling omits the second 'o' ('homeopathy') and there is increasing acceptance of this version; indeed it has to be employed if any benefit is to be gained from an internet search. As global communication is now so important, it seems appropriate in the 21st century to adopt this spelling.

such as codeine phosphate is antipathic, whereas the use of antibiotics for a bacterial enteritis is allopathic. Using a substance such as arsenic, which, when administered to a healthy individual is capable of producing diarrhoea, is an example of homeopathic medicine.

The Development of Modern Homeopathy

Not only are the Ancient Egyptians known to have treated illness using the homeopathic principle; the Ancient Greeks also refer to it. Hippocrates (*c*.460–*c*.375 BC) is quoted thus: 'The majority of maladies may be cured by the same things that have caused them.' Paracelsus (1493–1541), a physician born in what is now Switzerland, and one of the great medical figures of the era, proposed that medicines should be prescribed on the same basis. He was also a proponent of the 'Doctrine of Signatures', the ancient principle which states that the physical properties of a plant are an indication of its uses in medicine (for instance the dandelion, having a yellow flower, has a place in the treatment of jaundice). This doctrine remains as a tenet of modern day homeopathy. It was, however, not until the early 19th century that the system of homeopathy was fully developed, by a German physician by the name of Dr Christian Friedrich Samuel Hahnemann. Born in Saxony in 1755, he had received his medical degree from Erlangen University in 1779 but soon became disillusioned by the medical practices of the time, which he considered unscientific and barbaric. As a means of supporting himself and his family, Hahnemann turned to translating medical textbooks into German. While translating a text by a Scottish physician by the name of Cullen, he found himself disagreeing with the author's explanation of the mode of action of Peruvian Bark (Cinchona) in the treatment of 'Marsh Fever' (the disease we now know as malaria, and which was widespread in Europe at that time). Cullen asserted that the benefit was due to the 'tonic effect' of Cinchona on the stomach, but Hahnemann argued that while it was well known that some of the strongest 'tonics' had no effect on the disease, other medicines such as coffee and arsenic did so. There must be another reason why Cinchona bark could cure patients of this malady.

Always one to make his opinions known, Hahnemann actually wrote to Cullen to inform him of his opinion, but at the same time he set about experimenting on himself to investigate the phenomenon. He found that if he took a dose (four drachms) of Cinchona he experienced all the

2

physical symptoms of malaria, though without the actual fever. If he stopped taking the medicine, the symptoms gradually ceased, and if he recommenced dosing they reappeared. He concluded that the ability of Cinchona bark to relieve the symptoms of Marsh Fever depended on its ability to reproduce the symptoms when administered to a healthy individual. This he defined as the 'homeopathic effect', and Hahnemann devoted the rest of his life to developing a rational form of medicine, based on that principle. The *Cinchona experiment* was conducted in 1790. After a great deal more work, in 1796 he published an *Essay on a New Principle For Ascertaining The Curative Powers of Drugs, and Some Examination of the Previous Principles.*

The 'Law of Similars' he encapsulated in the phrase '*Similia similibus curentur*' – 'Let likes be cured by likes'. Thus armed, Hahnemann set about developing these principles in his practice, and spreading the word of this remarkable new form of medicine. A full description of the system was published in 1810 as *The Organon of the Medical Art.* Five further editions were to follow. The sixth edition was completed in 1842, but before it was printed, Hahnemann died, in Paris, on July 2nd 1843. He had been suffering from bronchitis for three months and was 88 years old.

His wife, Melanie, only made the existence of the manuscript known when other versions were claimed to be the sixth edition. She was committed to overseeing the publication herself in order to preserve Hahnemann's reputation, and the veracity of the text, but she too died before any of the several negotiations in which she participated could be completed. It then came into the hands of Melanie's adopted daughter Sophie, who had married into the family of von Boenning-hausen, a noted homeopath of the time, and of whom there is more information later in this chapter. It was from this family that the manuscript was eventually purchased, for US$1000, by Drs William Boericke and James William Ward. The sixth edition of the *Organon* was finally published in Germany in 1921, and in the USA in 1922.

The first three paragraphs of the *Organon* set the context for the practice of homeopathy and indeed of medicine itself, in whatever form. They are no less relevant to veterinary medicine:

§1

The physician's highest and *only* calling is to make the sick healthy, to cure, as it is called.

3

§2

The highest ideal of cure is the rapid, gentle and permanent restoration of health; that is, the lifting and annihilation of the disease in its entire extent in the shortest, most reliable, and least disadvantageous way, according to clearly realisable principles.

§3

To be a genuine practitioner of the medical art, a physician must:

- clearly realise what is to be cured in diseases, that is, in each single case of disease (*discernment of the disease*)
- clearly realise what is curative in medicines, that is, in each particular medicine (*knowledge of medicinal powers*)
- be aware of how to adapt what is curative in medicines to what he has discerned to be undoubtedly diseased in the patient, according to clear principles.

In this way, recovery must result.

Adapting what is curative in medicines to what is diseased in patients requires that the physician be able to:

- adapt the most appropriate medicine, according to its mode of action, to the case before him (*selection of the remedy*)
- prepare the medicine exactly as required
- give the medicine in the exact amount required (the right *dose*)
- properly time the repetition of doses.

Finally, the physician must know the obstacles to cure in each case and be aware of how to clear them away, so that the recovery of health may be permanent.

If the physician has this insight, discernment, knowledge and awareness then he understands how to act expediently and thoroughly, and he is a genuine practitioner of the medical art.

Provings

In order to accumulate the information on the medicines necessary to practice homeopathy, Hahnemann tested the effects of a large number of substances on healthy individuals, mostly members of his family, friends or students. He termed the collection of symptoms produced by the administration of a medicine to a healthy subject a 'Proving' (from the German 'Prüfung', meaning 'test'). The results of these experiments were published between 1811 and 1821 as his *Materia Medica Pura*. This work ran to three editions, the last of which was published in 1830 and contained accounts of 67 medicines.

Potentisation

Perhaps not surprisingly, Hahnemann found that the use of toxic medicines in the sick frequently caused a worsening of the patient's condition before the therapeutic effect appeared, and in an effort to reduce these effects he experimented with progressive dilutions of the medicines. Most of the work involved diluting the medicines one in a hundred at each stage (the 'centesimal' dilution scale). By meticulous experimentation, he discovered that, provided the dilution method involved vigorous shaking of each vial after each stage of dilution (a process now known as 'succussion'), the medicines not only became safer to use but also more powerful. His method of succussion was to beat the vials a preset number of times on a leather-bound book. As he considered that this process increased the energetic potential of the medicine he described it as 'dynamisation', but the process is now generally referred to as 'potentisation'.

The more stages of dilution and succussion a homeopathic remedy undergoes, the more potent it becomes. It is common nomenclature to consider potencies of 12th centesimal potency (12c) and below as 'low' potencies, and those above 12c as 'high'.

Totality

It also became obvious that the best results of treatment were obtained when the symptoms obtained from the provings of a medicine matched the complete symptomatology of the patient, not just the main presenting signs. Thus, if a patient presented for treatment of one group of symptoms, it was necessary to take into account any others from which that person was suffering. Such additional symptoms are known in homeopathy as 'concomitants', and the symptoms appertaining to the physical condition are known as 'local' (sometimes 'particular') symptoms. Furthermore, such symptoms as applied to the patient's general condition, such as appetite, craving for specific foods, and the effects of environmental conditions like heat, cold or changes in weather, also needed to be taken into account for a successful prescription. These symptoms, dealing as they do with the patient as a whole, are described as 'general' symptoms. Of even greater importance in the case-taking was an assessment of the mental and emotional state of the patient, the 'mental' symptoms. This concept of totality is vital to an understanding of homeopathy, as it sets disease in a holistic framework and concentrates on the individual patient and his symptoms, rather than on the named disease.

Chronic Disease

The latter part of Hahnemann's life was spent in contemplating chronic disease. He noticed that while patients would respond adequately to the homeopathic treatment of an acute disease state, often they would keep returning, either with the same symptoms, or different ones. His researches led him to postulate the miasmatic theory, whereby he suggested that chronic disease is due to the inherited or acquired potential to exhibit a particular pattern of disease. This is a complex and somewhat controversial area of homeopathy and is discussed in detail in subsequent chapters. However, Hahnemann revealed his thoughts on this when he published his second great philosophical work, *The Chronic Diseases, Their Peculiar Nature and Their Homeopathic Cure*, in 1828.

The Spread of Homeopathy

There is documentary evidence of Hahnemann's and his pupils' success in treating disease with homeopathy. In 1813, for instance, as Napoleon's army retreated from Moscow it met with Prussian troops at the Battle of Leipzig. The carnage resulted in a severe epidemic of typhus in the city. Hahnemann, resident in Leipzig at that time, cured 178 cases with only two fatalities. Eighteen years later, in the cholera epidemic of 1831, one of his pupils in Raab had only 6 fatalities (4%) from 154 patients treated, whereas in the same town, of 1500 patients treated by orthodox means, 55% died.

Clemens Maria Franz von Boenninghausen was born in Overssel, the Netherlands, in 1785. He studied law but as the owner of a large estate also had an interest in agriculture. In 1827 he was cured of tuberculosis by a student of Hahnemann and subsequently devoted his life to studying, practising and teaching homeopathy. It was his son Karl who married Sophie Hahnemann. Among his most famous works are *The Therapeutic Pocketbook* and the voluminous *Characteristics*.

Homeopathy was introduced to Great Britain in 1832 by Frederick Foster Hervey Quin (1799–1878), who had visited Hahnemann in Leipzig. Quin helped to established the first homeopathic hospital, in Soho, later to become the Royal London Homoeopathic Hospital, which is still in operation to this day within the aegis of the National Health Service. In 1854 there was a cholera epidemic in London: the mortality at the Homoeopathic Hospital was 16%, compared to a rate of 52% at the orthodox hospitals. Interestingly, these figures were suppressed by the health authorities of the time, and it was only after much pressure that they were discussed in Parliament and admitted to the official report.

Constantine Hering (1800–1880) was a pupil of Hahnemann who introduced homeopathy into the USA when he settled there in 1833. Perhaps his most famous achievement was the formulation of 'Hering's Law', the observation that after homeopathic treatment the resolution of a patient's symptoms follows a recognisable pattern. (This is discussed more fully in Chapter 4.) Hering also proved a large number of new medicines, including the South American bushmaster snake (*Lachesis muta*), and was the author of *Guiding Symptoms of our Materia Medica* (1879–1891), a distinct change in direction in the way materia medica was presented in that it relied more heavily on clinical experience than provings.

In late 19th century England, Richard Hughes (1836–1902) and his predecessor Robert Ellis Dudgeon (1820–1904) dominated homeopathic thinking, being highly sceptical of the high potency prescribing used by Hahnemann in his later life (and further developed by Kent and his associates in the USA). Hughes relied exclusively on low potency medicines, matched by materia medica based on toxic drug symptoms alone. This philosophy lives on in the form of the low potency remedies frequently dispensed to the present day in continental Europe.

By contrast, the American physician J.T. Kent (1849–1916) is considered to be the father of high potency prescribing and developed the use of very high potencies such as 1M (1000c) and beyond. Kent also expanded the concept of the 'repertory', a lexicon of symptoms with a list of medicines which are known to be indicated for each one, as a key to the materia medica. Hahnemann himself had compiled such a work (*Fragmenta de Viribus Medicamentorum Positivis*, 1805) and in 1834 one of his pupils, George Jahr (1800–1875), published his *Manual* as a repertory to Hahnemann's work. Boenninghausen had published his own *Repertory of the Anti-Psoric Remedies* in 1833. However,

Kent's repertory was far more detailed and easier to use and for decades remained the standard. He originally compiled it for his own use, but he was persuaded by his pupils to make it more widely available. It was initially published section by section, and only later was the work compiled into a single volume. For many years the standard work of its type, it forms the basis of most of the modern computer repertories.

Just as important as his work on the repertory, however, was Kent's presentation of the materia medica. Along with many of his contemporaries, Kent was heavily influenced by the philosophy of Emmanuel Swedenborg (1688–1772), a Swedish scientist who attempted to incorporate theology into rational science; in consequence, Kent's *Lectures on Homeopathic Philosophy* provides a philosophical view of disease bordering on the spiritual. His *Lectures on Materia Medica*, written in an easy narrative style, introduces the idea of a 'picture' of the remedy – when this picture is grasped it is easy to remember and recognise in a patient. Vital to conceptualising this 'remedy picture' is a knowledge of the mental and emotional state associated with the remedy, and Kent laid great emphasis on Hahnemann's assertion in paragraph 211 of the *Organon* that the mental symptoms, being the most characteristic of the patient, are of paramount importance in selecting the appropriate remedy. This concept has now been developed further by modern workers such as Vithoulkas and Sankaran.

The history of homeopathy in the USA in the 20th century is one of decline and resurgence. In the late 19th century, the homeopathic colleges gradually incorporated orthodox medicine into their curricula, and medical practitioners were encouraged to use allopathic diagnosis and treatment methods, incorporating low potency homeopathic remedies as only one part of an overall stratagem. Those few homeopaths who continued to follow the philosophy of Hahnemann and Kent became increasingly isolated and by 1940, of the 23 homeopathic colleges operating in the 1890s only one remained; by 1958 there were none. The split between 'low potency' homeopathic prescribers and 'high potency' prescribers, together with the advent of modern drugs such as antibiotics hastened the decline; in addition, various political moves within the medical profession ensured that the decline in homeopathy in the USA was dramatic, to say the least. Happily, a resurgence in interest in the late 20th century occurred and homeopathy in the USA is now again undergoing rapid development, with some of the world's leading homeopaths residing there.

In the UK a similar though less dramatic fall from favour was experienced, but homeopathy retained a significant place in medicine throughout the early twentieth century, and workers such as Dr Margaret Blackie carried the torch. Royal patronage must certainly have been an important factor in this, but the survival of homeopathic hospitals in London, Bristol, Glasgow, and Tunbridge Wells, and a thriving Outpatients at Liverpool, owes more to the efficacy of their methods than to politics.

After the launching of the British National Health Service in 1948, homeopathy was given official status in 1950 with the formation by Act of Parliament of the Faculty of Homeopathy. The Faculty was established to oversee the training and practice of homeopathic doctors and for many years ran the only training courses available to medical practitioners. However, with the emergence of an increasing number of teaching centres, it has in recent years ceased to be directly involved in teaching and instead performs regulatory and accreditation functions.

In parallel with the development of medical homeopathy, non-medically qualified practitioners (NMQPs) have practised homeopathy in the UK since its introduction. While receiving no officially recognised medical training, many of the world's leading homeopathic thinkers have emerged from the ranks of the NMQPs and at present there is a move to provide some kind of official recognition and control of this large body of practitioners.

From its origins in Europe, homeopathy spread throughout the globe, and there are few countries in the world where it is not practised in one form or another. Sometimes it was introduced by a formally-trained doctor, but often it was a lay practitioner who sowed the seeds of homeopathy. For instance it was an Indian businessman who, around the middle of the 19th century, encouraged his doctor to investigate homeopathy and thus instigated the practice of homeopathy on that sub-continent. Today there are 110 institutes teaching homeopathy in India, all attached to universities, and approximately 150,000 homeopathic practitioners. The first person to practice homeopathy in Australia was probably Mr Thienette de Bergny, a lay practitioner in Victoria around 1850, but Dr John Hickson appears to have been the first homeopathic doctor, practising in Melbourne around the same time.

Veterinary Homeopathy

Veterinary homeopathy has a history almost as long as that of its medical counterpart. Hahnemann himself treated animals and indeed delivered a lecture on the subject to the Leipzig Economic Society in about 1813; the manuscript now resides in the Universitätsbibliothek at Leipzig.

Von Boenninghausen used homeopathy on the animals of his country estate in what is now northern Germany. However the 'father' of veterinary homeopathy is generally considered to be Joseph Lux (1773–1849), a German veterinary surgeon, who published Volume I of his *Zooiasis or Homeopathy in its Application to the Diseases of Animals* in 1837. It was also he who pioneered the use of isopathy (see page 138) with his work on anthrax in cattle.

In the UK James Moore (1807–1886), a Scottish veterinary surgeon, championed homeopathy within the veterinary profession. A member of the Council of the Royal College of Veterinary Surgeons from 1873 to 1877, he was a prolific author, writing several books and pamphlets during his lifetime. Among these were *Outlines of Veterinary Homoeopathy* (ten editions published between 1857 and 1899), *Diseases of Dogs and their Homoeopathic Treatment* (seven editions between 1863 and 1870, and reprinted in 1991 by B.Jain in India), and *Horses Ill and Well, Homoeopathic Treatment* (five editions between 1873 and 1885).

Many other books on veterinary homeopathy survive from the 19th century, for instance *Elements of Veterinary Homoeopathy* (1852) written by W. Haycock, a veterinary surgeon who qualified at Edinburgh and practised in Huddersfield, Yorkshire. In the USA, F.E. Boericke's *Homeopathic Veterinary Practice* was published in 1874. Again in the UK, 15,000 copies of Dr Ruddock's *Pocket Manual of Homoeopathic Veterinary Medicine* were printed, and *The Homoeopathic Telephone* published in Tasmania in 1883 states that 'every farmer and stockowner should possess the *Veterinary Vade Mecum* edited by Messrs Rush and Lord, MRCVS Eng.'

However, despite having been such an integral part of veterinary medicine for so long, it appears that veterinary homeopathy in the UK had all but died out by the 1950s. Fortunately, a few veterinary surgeons continued to practice it, notable among them being Ken Biddis and George Macleod. Biddis published a small booklet entitled *Homoeopathy in Veterinary Practice* as support for the staff of the People's

Dispensary for Sick Animals. At that time, this charity trained its own practitioners, and as such the use of prescription drugs was precluded. Homeopathy provided a cheap and effective form of medicine which was ideal for such an organisation. A second edition of Biddis' booklet was published in 1987.

George Macleod used homeopathy extensively in his mixed practice in the north of Scotland, and subsequently in Sussex, and in 1977 he published *The Homoeopathic Treatment of Horses*, to be followed later by volumes on other species. Macleod was a key figure in the survival of veterinary homeopathy in the post-war era and a major force in the regeneration of interest in this form of therapy in the profession in the 1970s. His books remain as a body of work of international significance.

Another current major influence is Chris Day, who was exposed to homeopathy by a family connection with his uncle, a homeopathic doctor in Germany. Chris's mother used homeopathy in the family veterinary practice in Oxfordshire and Chris has practised homeopathy from the day of his qualification in 1972. The publication of *The Homoeopathic Treatment of Small Animals* in 1984 remains a landmark in veterinary homeopathy. He followed this in 1995 with *The Homoeopathic Treatment of Beef and Dairy Cattle*.

Francis Hunter was introduced to homeopathy after meeting the family doctor of a farmer friend and subsequently studied on the Faculty of Homeopathy medical courses. Along with Day, Macleod and one of the authors (J.S.) he lectured on the first veterinary courses at the Faculty. In 1984 he published *Homeopathic First Aid Treatment for Pets*, the four editions of which sold nearly 30,000 copies. His most recent book, *Everyday Homeopathy for Animals*, was published in 2004.

Macleod, Hunter and Day were instrumental in the foundation in 1982 of the British Association of Homeopathic Veterinary Surgeons and it was due primarily to Chris Day's work with the Faculty of Homeopathy that in 1984 the veterinary course at the Royal London Homeopathic Hospital was established, perhaps the first such course in the world. This was followed in 1987 by the awarding of the first veterinary qualification, the Veterinary Membership of the Faculty of Homeopathy. At the time of writing there are 49 such qualified veterinary surgeons and the number increases every year. These include four Veterinary Fellows of the Faculty, the Fellowship being awarded for outstanding contributions to veterinary homeopathy.

In 2001, a Primary Certificate in Veterinary Homeopathy was developed, both as an opportunity for those not wishing to pursue their study to full Membership, and also as a first step to the latter. There are now three veterinary teaching centres in UK accredited by the Faculty of Homeopathy: the Homeopathic Professionals Teaching Group (HPTG) based in Oxford, and the Bristol and Glasgow Homeopathic Hospitals. The HPTG currently also run courses in Australia and the Republic of Ireland.

The spread of veterinary homeopathy around the world has mirrored that of medical homeopathy and it is practised in over 30 countries. In the USA, Dr Richard Pitcairn graduated from veterinary school in 1965. Dissatisfied with the results of orthodox treatment in his patients he returned to academia to study microbiology for a PhD degree. However, he still 'did not know any better how to cure disease'. This led him to study the role of nutrition in disease, and subsequently to investigate homeopathy; in 1996 he co-founded the Academy of Veterinary Homeopathy to provide professional course training and an entity for certification purposes.

Don Hamilton developed an interest in homeopathy in the search for a more successful way of managing chronic disease and in 1999 published *Homeopathic Care for Cats and Dogs*, the most comprehensive work of its type to date.

Elsewhere, regulated courses in veterinary homeopathy now exist in several countries, among them Austria, Germany, Italy and Hungary.

Significant publications on veterinary homeopathy in non-English languages include: *Omeopatica veterinaria* (del Francia 1985), *Bewährte Indikationen der Homöopathie in der Veterinärmedizin* (Rakow, B. and Rakow, M. 1988), *Kompendium der Tierärztlichen Homöopathie* (Wolter, H. 1989) and *Veterinaer homøopati* (Brock, K. and Nielsen, J. 1986).

The International Association for Veterinary Homeopathy (IAVH) was formed in 1986. It holds a biennial conference and awards a Certificate of Veterinary Homeopathy, attainable after completion of an accredited course of education, followed by written and practical examinations. The Association's Education Committee was formed in 1997 and is responsible for IAVH accreditation of tutors and courses in veterinary homeopathy.

Homeopathy has a long and fascinating history, with no small amount of romance and intrigue, and its development owes much to the passion and sheer dogged hard work of a number of dedicated doctors, veterinary surgeons and non-medically qualified homeopaths around the world. For those with a penchant for the human and political side of medicine, accounts of Hahnemann's life and of the demise of homeopathy in the USA make interesting reading. Veterinary homeopathy itself has mirrored and often contributed to the developments in human homeopathy and stands today in a position of opportunity unparalleled in its history. The increasing demand of the animal owner for homeopathy bodes for an exciting and enormously satisfying future for its practitioners.

References

Hahnemann, C.F.S. (1996) *Organon of the Medical Art* (translated from *The Organon*, 6th edn, 1842 by Stephen Decker and edited by Wenda Brewster O'Reilly). Redmond: Birdcage Books.

Schofield, D. (2004) The father of British homeopathy? *Annual Conference of the British Association of Homeopathic Veterinary Surgeons.*

Winston, J. (1999) *The Faces of Homeopathy.* Tawa, New Zealand: Great Auk Publishing.

Yasgur, J. (1998) *Homeopathic Dictionary and Holistic Health Reference* (4th edn). Greenville, PA: Van Hoy Publishers.

Chapter 2

Research into Homeopathy

How *Can* It Work?

One 'fact' that is widely quoted about homeopathy is that its basis is the giving of remedies in an extremely diluted form. It must, of course, be remembered that the fundamental homeopathic principle of 'likes curing likes' has nothing to do with dilution. However, dilution is widely regarded as being integral to the method and for some this is enough to damn the whole discipline out of hand, on the basis that the dilutions are so great that they cannot possibly have any effect. The argument has even been seriously advanced that since it is known that homeopathy can't work, there is no point in wasting any time trying to prove that it does, as any proof that does emerge must by definition be wrong!

It is true that one of the biggest obstacles to the acceptance of homeopathy is the concept of the ultra-high dilutions. The magical 'Avogadro's number' is often quoted, this being the point beyond which, according to Newtonian principles, it can be shown both mathematically and experimentally that not one single molecule of the original substance remains. This represents a dilution of 6.023×10 to the power of minus 23, and this is reached at around the 24x or 12c potencies (see Chapter 3 for details of potency). The majority of treatments utilise potencies considerably beyond this point.

The question of trial work will be discussed below but, that apart, medical minds seem to stick on this question of dilution. This is perhaps understandable, given that for most of them the main area of interest is clinical. However, during the 20th century, and especially during the latter half, the scientific world generally began to realise that the concepts of Newtonian physics, whilst still retaining much validity, could not provide the necessary framework to explain and explore the newer phenomena that were being identified in the natural world. Accordingly, newer disciplines such as quantum physics, quantum mechanics and quantum biology came into being, and these have revolutionised our understanding of the nature of matter and its relationship to energy. In these newer disciplines the principles that are the necessary prerequisites for homeopathy to work are readily accepted, on both a theoretical and an experimental level. While the particular mechanisms involved in homeopathy have not been absolutely defined experimentally, from considerations of these new concepts, biophysical models have been devised that not only account for its action on a theoretical basis but also predict the same requirements for the practical application of the method that Hahnemann laid down over 200 years ago (Poitevin 1995: Towsey, Hasan 1995). These and other models draw on ideas such as chaos theory, morphic and stochastic resonance and the quantum coherence in liquids. The paradoxes in the known physical microscopic nature and behaviour of water can also be explained by these theories. Studies on the behaviour of ethanol/water systems (Singh and Chabra 1993) have shown the feasibility of the energy transference and storage required by homeopathy, as well as accounting for changes in the structure and properties of the water involved in remedy dilutions beyond Avogadro's number (Bourkas 1996; Elia 2004). (See Chapter 3 for a discussion of the process of succussion.)

The work of Benveniste using the Human Basophil Degranulation Test published in *Nature* (1988) showed that the degranulation reaction could be triggered by anti-immunoglobulins at dilutions in the ultramolecular range. The subsequent debunking of this work using a professional magician and similar methods of doubtful scientific validity, and the associated attack on the concept of the 'memory of water', represent a controversial period in the history of homeopathic research. However, work of a similar nature at Queen's University Belfast by Professor Ennis, and repeated at four independent universities in France, Italy, Belgium, and Holland (Belon et al 1999) has subsequently shown his basic findings to be valid. Professor Ennis herself performed the experiment twice (Brown and Ennis 2001). It is interesting to note that this latter work was instigated and co-ordinated through Queen's University in an attempt to provide a truly scientific evaluation of Benveniste's work, with the expectation that it would be found wanting. The fact that his work was both validated and shown to be independently reproducible may well prove to be highly significant for basic research into homeopathy (Belon 2004; Fisher 2004).

Experiments in both humans and animals have demonstrated that ultra-high dilutions do produce measurable physiological effects, and also that the degree of the effects produced varies in direct proportion to the dilution (Nirmal 1987). Cholesterol and serum globulin levels have been shown to be affected by the remedy Chelidonium (Vakil, Vakil and Nanabhai 1989; Baumans et al 1987), and anti-inflammatory activity has been linked to homeopathic preparations of Arnica, Hypericum and Silica (Desai et al 1992). Baptisia as mother tincture can induce leukopoenia in rabbits (Engineer, Valik and Engineer 1990). The remedies Arsenicum Album, Bismuth and Plumbum have all produced increased elimination of the respective metal in cases of poisoning (Cazin et al 1991; Lapp, Wurmster, Ney 1955; Bukhsh 1999). Homeopathic Phosphorus, which is used clinically in cases where there is liver destruction, has proved able in the laboratory to protect against artificially induced hepatic damage (Guillemain 1987). Similar activity has been demonstrated using dexamethasone in potency to inhibit the action of the drug in its material form (Bonamin 2001).

Homeopathy maintains that there is a difference between a straight dilution and a potentised remedy (Chapter 3). Basic biological research measuring the effect of homeopathic thyroxine in various dilutions on the development of the common frog has verified that claim (Endler et al 1991), and it has also been confirmed with experiments on wheat and oat germination (Bornoroni 1991). Histamine in succussed ultra-dilutions has been shown to significantly affect the development and resolution of inflammation under experimental conditions, while similar dilutions of zinc have been used to influence the production of histamine in rats (Conforti et al 1993; Harish and Kretschmer 1988).

There have been many more studies carried out over the years which confirm the fact that ultra-diluted, succussed solutions are capable of producing a physiological effect. Many have been published in the *British Journal of Homeopathy* (now called *Homeopathy*), and some in conventional physiological journals. From them, and those cited above, two effects emerge which are vital for the functioning of homeopathy. The first is that forms of the same substance that are either undiluted or ultra-diluted with succussion can both have a specific effect on the same organ or system. The second is that the ultra-dilution changes the effect that is observed using the same substance in undiluted form. These findings are in complete accord with the principle which is recognised in the conventional medical field and known as the Arndt-Schultz law. Also known as hormesis, or the biphasic response, this has demon-strated that in biological systems a small stimulus will encourage growth, a moderate one slows it and/or maintains the status quo, while a strong challenge inhibits activity. The term hormesis is generally used for the growth stimulant effects of small quantities of toxic material (Robinson 1992).

Thus both theoretical considerations and practical experiments demonstrate the fact that homeopathy *can* work. In the clinical field both controlled trials and other studies provide ample evidence that it *does* work.

Clinical Trials and Their Problems

The use of the double-blind trial is for many with a conventional scientific training the ultimate benchmark for determining efficacy, and it is not generally realised that the first use of the blinding method came from the homeopathic world. In 1879, due to concerns about the placebo effect during provings, a blind technique was employed by a homeopathic group in a homeopathic trial sponsored by the Milwaukee Academy of Medicine and reported in the New York *Homeopathic Times* in March 1880 (Kaptchuk 1997). The remedy concerned was Aconite in a 30c potency. The first use of the technique in conventional medicine appears to have been in psychology by Pierce and Jastrow in 1883, and its major acceptance was in 1938 with a trial involving the use of sulphonamides in pneumonia. In contrast, homeopathic circles were using the technique as routine in provings from 1900. With its emphasis on randomisation, blinding of the investigators to prevent bias, adequate control groups, and cross-over of treatment groups, its usefulness cannot be denied although the method as it has developed does have its limitations, and these are now being increasingly recognised even within conventional medicine. Its limitations when applied to homeopathy are greater for a number of reasons but it can still yield useful data.

A major difficulty is that in most cases a homeopathic medicine is prescribed on the basis of the characteristics of the individual patient, with account being taken of all the subtle differences that are found between all individuals. In contrast, the great principle of the clinical trial is standardisation. If the prescription of the remedy being investigated is based on a pathological indication, e.g. Arnica in bruising, then the method holds, but if the circumstances are such that different homeopathic remedies would be given to different patients for the same conventionally-named condition, then it falls apart in its pure form. To be meaningful, the protocol and the interpretation must be modified to take account of the homeopathic method. It is at this point that homeo-pathy is often accused of 'moving the goalposts', whereas in fact all that is being asked is that a realistic account is taken of the homeopathic method. It is possible to apply the double-blind technique to homeopathy provided the essential difference between the prescribing methods is acknowledged and built into the design of the trial. However, if the conventional design is insisted on, then the results will not be valid, as like will not be compared with like.

The conventional medical approach begins by defining a named condition and then devising a treatment for it. Thus Mr/Mrs X is diagnosed as suffering from arthritis and treatment is on the basis of that diagnosis. Homeopathy begins by considering Mr/Mrs X as a whole person, including the fact that they suffer from arthritis (see Chapter 6 for a deeper discussion of this point). This means that, whereas all conventional patients would be given the same anti-inflammatory treatment, it does not follow that all homeopathic patients would neces-sarily receive the same remedy.

In a trial involving a drug and a homeopathic remedy, using a conventional protocol, randomly selected groups would be compared with each other and against a common assessment of response. But while all participants would be considered suitable cases for treat-ment with the conventional drug, not all the homeopathically treated patients would necessarily be similarly suited to the same remedy. One assessment for inclusion in a trial involving Rhus Toxicodendron found that 58% of those willing to participate were not in fact suitable for treatment with the remedy (Fisher, Greenwood and Huskisson 1989).

The process of randomisation poses other considerations, although these are more applicable to the human field than the veterinary. The ethics of the human situation dictate that all participants in a trial shall be volunteers. This will necessarily exclude certain people who prefer, for a variety of reasons, not to be 'guinea-pigs'. From the homeopathic point of view this will exclude certain mental types, since the mental picture will always, wherever possible, form an important part of any homeopathic prescription.

All these considerations can easily be taken into account, and doing so results in very different interpretations. A trial involving the remedy Baryta Carbonica for the treatment of hypertension, which analysed the results in two different ways, demonstrates this fact. Analysis of the results in the conventional manner produced no significant difference

18

between the groups. However, all patients in the homeopathically treated group had been independently assessed as to their suitability for the treatment, and when this was taken into account there was a statistically significant result in favour of homeopathy (Bignamini et al 1987).

A further refinement of the basic trial technique poses more problems for homeopathy. This is the cross-over procedure. Homeopathic remedies may have their effect over considerable periods of time, and on occasion the onset of their action may be delayed, only starting after the cross-over has occurred. This means that a group that has received a homeopathic treatment initially cannot with any validity be given a conventional drug later in the trial. The slower onset of action of homeopathic remedies as compared with conventional medications will also have implications for the time scale over which the results of trials are assessed. The faster-acting conventional medication may erroneously appear superior to the homeopathic remedy if short-term assessment is the only criterion used, whereas a longer-term review may reveal a slower onset but better maintained response in favour of the homeopathic remedy. The immune status of the participants in a trial can also, in certain circumstances, potentially affect the response to homeopathy more than to conventional medication.

Some of the above may not appear to be directly applicable to veterinary homeopathy. However, the validation of the homeopathic method is not confined to one area only. The problems associated with the obtaining of valid research results are common to all species and the constraints encountered in one field are often applicable in another.

There are a number of reasons why the practicability of a controlled trial may need to be reconsidered. It may be realised that the methodology is not in fact suitable for an accurate assessment of homeopathy. Another reason may be ethical considerations. One such interesting case in Mexico involved a blind trial using Phosphorus for the treatment of rectal prolapse in pigs. The supervising veterinary surgeon, who had been at first a reluctant and sceptical participant, refused after a while, on humane grounds, to allow the trial to continue. His reason was that the benefits of the homeopathic treatment were demonstrably so great that it was unethical to deprive the control group of the benefits of that treatment (Searcy and Guajardo 1994)!

Other trial work in the veterinary field has demonstrated the value of homeopathy. Blind trials involving the use of nosodes (Chapter 11) have shown benefit in the treatment of bovine mastitis. In a 40-cow milking herd, split randomly into two equal groups, the incidence of mastitis in the treatment group was reduced from 47.5% to 2.5%. Corresponding improvements were also seen in cell count levels. Administration of the remedy was via the drinking water. There was no significant change in the recovery time for those clinical cases that did occur (Day 1986). Similar work in Mexico using the remedies Conium, Phosphorus and Phytolacca produced a reduction in clinical mastitis from 42.8% to 7.1% (p<0.05) (Searcy and Guajardo 1994). The trial involved 26 beasts in two groups of 13. The picture in relation to subclinical mastitis was similarly improved in another trial. Both trials used the Californian Mastitis Test as the assessment method. (Searcy, Reyes and Guajardo 1995).

The use of homeopathy as a growth promoter in pigs has been investigated in two placebo-controlled blind trials, both with statistically significant outcomes in favour of homeopathy, which could not be accounted for merely by an appetite stimulant effect. One involved the use of Sulphur 200c in pregnant sows (Guarjardo 1996), the other the administration of Baryta Carbonicum LM1 to piglets with retarded growth (Briones 1989).

A blind trial in humans has demonstrated the efficacy of using Caulophyllum as an aid to labour (Eid et al) and these results have been reproduced with cattle, pigs and bitches in repeated studies (Day 1985, 1984; Grandmontagne 1995). In all species there were significant reductions in the time required for parturition, with a corresponding reduction in the associated stress. Day (1984) has used Caulophyllum in a herd of 130 sows where the rate of stillbirths was 20%. Management, dietary and infectious causes had been eliminated, as had boar fertility. The initial trial involved 20 sows in two groups of 10, one group receiving treatment with the other acting as a control. Caulophyllum 30c was administered twice weekly for three weeks before farrowing. Using the Fischer probability test there was a statistically significant result in favour of the treated group. Following this result the whole herd was treated with the remedy and piglet mortality overall fell to 2.6%. After six months the treatment was stopped and in two months the mortality rose to 14.9%. Treatment was recommenced and the mortality fell once more to 1.9%. Porcine Mastitis/Metritis/Agalactia complex has been the object of a positively significant trial using Phytolacca, and similar work has been undertaken in humans (Richter 1999). Sepia has been the subject of a trial in dairy cattle involving 120 animals divided into 4 random groups being given various combinations of remedy and placebo. All the parameters of holding to service, calving interval and calving percentage in a commercial herd situation have shown a statistically significant improvement following the use of the remedy (Williamson et al 1991, 1995).

A pilot study using a double-blind protocol has produced encouraging results in respect of the combination of Arsenicum Album and conventional medication in the treatment of neonatal diarrhoea in calves (Kayne and Rafferty 1994). A similar double-blind trial involving diarrhoea in children gave statistically significant results in favour of homeopathy. The methodology of the trial took account of the individual nature of homeopathic prescribing, with a variety of remedies being used according to the individual clinical symptoms (Jacobs et al 1994).

Other Research Approaches

As indicated above, the blind trial, while being a useful tool, has its disadvantages. Also, total reliance on it means that much valuable information that is available from the clinical situation is not being utilised. This is true no matter what system of medicine is being considered, and hence the development of additional techniques such as epidemiological studies, randomised comparative studies and clinical audit. In epidemic situations, 'before and after studies' are also of value. While improved standardisation of the protocols for these approaches will increase the validity of the results, those already achieved give strong evidence of the efficacy of homeopathy. Canine tracheobronchitis and distemper outbreaks in kennels have both been the subject of successful 'before and after' studies involving nosodes, with the incidence of disease being reduced by 97.9% and 62.6% respectively, the latter involving a study of some 13,000 dogs over 3 years (Day 1987; Saxton 1991). A similar type of study on calves being transported abroad for slaughter gave comparable results using Nux Vomica, the parameters here being associated with journey recovery time and subsequent carcass quality (Mahe 1987).

A comparative study between individually selected homeopathic remedies and medroxyprogesterone injections in the treatment of house soiling in cats yielded a statistically significant result in favour of homeopathy (Knaff 2000). Both this study and that involving tracheobronchitis demonstrated an interesting additional aspect, in that evidence emerged that previous conventional treatment could have an adverse effect on the efficacy of subsequent homeopathic therapy. Dogs that had received the intra-nasal vaccine against *Bordetella bronchiseptica* showed a decreased response to the subsequently administered nosode compared to others that had not received the vaccine, while cats having had prior conventional treatment also showed a decreased response to subsequent homeopathic treatment.

A study of Cushing's disease in dogs and horses using a standardised homeopathic approach has indicated an 80% excellent response rate with remission of clinical symptoms. 10% gave a poor response and 10% had no response at all (Elliott 2001). Many of these animals had previously received conventional treatment with no comparable effect.

Clinical audit is being used increasingly in the human field, and various protocols have been devised and are in use. The technique involves the use of patient questionnaires to assess the subjective responses to treatment, as well as objective assessments where appropriate. Case records may also be utilised in the process, either on their own or in conjunction with other sources. Grading of response is within pre-set parameters ranging from excellent to worse, thus allowing unified interpretations to be made (Heger 2001). These methods show very positive results for homeopathy generally. Parts of the assessment involve subjective judgements by the patient, and hence some aspects of the approach will require modification for the veterinary field. Subjective assessments by the owner of the animal may well be applicable, but with appropriate modifications the method is intrinsically valid for both disciplines.

An overall assessment of research can be obtained by using meta-analysis, whereby previously published results are collectively measured against a minimum set standard of methodology. All studies falling below that standard are excluded, so that the combined results reflect the best of the trial work available. A number of these studies have been done in relation to homeopathy (Bol 1998; Kleijnen, Knipschild and ter Riet 1991; Linde 1994, 1998). All were carried out by conventional workers and analysed using conventional techniques, and all have been favourable to homeopathy.

Homeopathic research is often criticised for the poor quality of its methodology. Although there are undoubtedly faults in individual trials, one finding of meta-analysis has been that overall the level of error is no greater than that generally found in the conventional field.

The Future

It is sometimes claimed that homeopathy is not willing to subject itself to critical analysis. The above overview, although brief, will have indicated that this is untrue. Much research has been carried out and the subject continues to be investigated at all levels. Modern research is increasingly bridging the gap between homeopathy and conventional medicine, and much conventional research in the field of immunology is providing independent support for homeopathy (Grange and Denman 1993). The reader is referred to the book *The Emerging Science of Homeopathy* (Bellavite and Signorini) for further details of this. It has also been established that results are reproducible (Reilly 1994) and, in laboratory conditions, not confined to mammals (Bastide 1994; Youbicier-Simo 1993).

While there is no doubt that more research work needs to be done, enough has already been achieved to demonstrate beyond reasonable doubt that homeopathy as a therapeutic method is valid. However, the protocols for research must be geared to the realities of the therapy if truly meaningful results are to be obtained. That is not to imply that there should be any relaxation of scientific rigour, but rather to recognise that the search for genuine scientific truth cannot be confined to one rigid set of rules, and to apply evenly such rigour as is desirable. It could be argued that, if the conditions of proof required from homeopathy were as rigorously applied to all medical procedures, then at least 50% of the tried and trusted procedures of conventional medicine would be banned overnight!

There is much discussion concerning the nature of the placebo response and its effect on the outcome of trials. Many in the medical homeopathic world will quote the positive results in animals as overwhelming evidence for homeopathy on the grounds that there can be no placebo response with animals. This may not be entirely true, especially in the companion animal sphere where there is a close emotional and energetic link between owner and pet. However, one fruitful way forward is to utilise research methods that compare two or more types of treatment directly rather than comparing each against the standard of the placebo. This approach is already being advocated by some in the conventional world and has much to recommend it.

But homeopathy is not an abstract science, it is a practical therapeutic method. The principle claims of homeopathy have been adequately demonstrated and explained by basic research, with a number of feasible models being postulated. While work on these must continue, the major way forward for research should be primarily in the clinical situation, not in the laboratory, for the ultimate test of any therapeutic system is a cured patient.

References

Bastide, M. et al. (1985) Activity and chronopharmacology of very low doses of physiological immunc inducers. *Immunology Today* **6**, 234.

Baumans, V. et al. (1987) Does Chelidonium 3x lower serum cholesterol? *British Homeopathic Journal* **76**, 14.

Bellavite, P. and Signorini, A. (2002) *The Emerging Science of Homeopathy*. Berkeley, CA: North Atlantic Books.

Belon, P. et al. (1999) Inhibition of human basophil degranulation by successive histamine dilutions: results of a European multi-centre trial. *Inflammation Research* **48** (Suppl. 1), S17-S18.

Belon, P. et al. (2004) Histamine dilutions modulate basophil activity. *Inflammation Research* **53**, 181-188.

Benveniste. J. (1988) Basophil degranulation in relation to increasing dilutions of anti-IgE antibody. *Nature* **333**, 816–818.

Bignamini, M. et al. (1987) Controlled double blind trial with Baryta Carb. 15c versus placebo in hypertensive patients. *British Homeopathic Journal* **76**, 114.

Bol, A. (1998) New meta-analysis of randomised controlled trials in homeopathy: efficacy of homeopathy is more than placebo effect. *Homint R&D Newsletter* 1/98.

Bonamin, L.V. et al. (2002) Very high dilutions of dexamethasone inhibit its pharmacological effects in vivo. *British Homeopathic Journal* **90**, 198-203.

Bornoroni, C. (1991) Synergism of action between indoleacetic acid and highly diluted solutions of $CaCO_2$ on the growth of oat coleoptiles. *Berlin Journal of Research Homeopathy* **1**(4-5), 275.

Bourkas, P. (1996) The measurements of the homeopathic remedies. *European Journal of Classical Homeopathy* **1**, 34.

Briones, F. (1989) Effect of Barium Carb., Calcium Carb., and Calcium Phosphoricum on the weight of pigs with retarded growth. *International Journal for Veterinary Homeopathy* **4**, 2; *British Homeopathic Journal* (2002) **89**(2).

Brown, V. and Ennis, M. (2001) Flow-cytometric analysis of basophil activation: inhibition by histamine at conventional and homeopathic concentrations. *Inflammation Research* **50** (Suppl. 2), 47–48.

Cazin, J. et al. (1991) Study of the effects of decimal and centesimal dilutions of arsenic on the retentions and mobilisation of arsenic in the rat. *Human Toxicology* **6**, 315.

Conforti, A. et al. (1993) Effects of high dilutions of histamine and other natural compounds on acute inflammation in rats. *Omeomed* **92**. Editrice compositori Bologna 163.

Day, C.E.I. (1984) Control of stillbirths using homeopathy. *Veterinary Record* **114**, 216.

Day, C.E.I. (1985) Clinical trials in bovine mastitis using Dystocia prevention. *Proceedings of LMHI Congress*, Lyon.

Day, C.E.I. (1986) Nosodes for prevention. *International Journal of Veterinary Homeopathy* **1**, 15.

Day, C.E.I. (1987) Isopathic prevention of kennel cough. *International Journal of Veterinary Homeopathy* **2**, 57.

Desai, V. et al. (1992) Anti-inflammatory activity of Arnica on rat paw oedema. *Third IAVH Congress*, Munster, Germany.

Eid, P. et al. (1993) Applicability of homeopathic Caulophyllum during labour. *British Homeopathic Journal* **82**, 245.

Elia et al. (2004) Permanent physico-chemical properties of extremely diluted solutions of homeopathic remedies. *Homeopathy* **93**(3), 144–150.

Elliot, M. (2001) Cushing's disease. A new approach to therapy in equine and canine patients. *British Homeopathic Journal* **90**(1).

Endler, P. et al. (1991) Effects of highly diluted succussed Thyroxine on metamorphosis of highland frogs. *Berlin Journal of Research into Homeopathy* **1**(3), 151.

Engineer, S., Vakil, S. and Engineer, L. (1990) A study of antibody formation by Baptista tinctoria mother tincture in experimental animals. *British Homeopathic Journal* **79**, 109.

Fisher, P., Greenwood, A. and Huskinsson, E.C. (1989) Effect of homeopathic treatment on fibrositis. *British Medical Journal* August.

Fisher, P. (2004) A landmark for basic research in homeopathy. *Homeopathy* **93**(3).

Grange, J. and Denman, A. (1993) Microdose-mediated immune modulation: a possible key to a scientific re-evaluation of homeopathy. *British Homeopathic Journal* **82**, 113.

Guajardo-Bernal, G. et al. (1996) Growth promoting effect of Sulphur 201c in pigs. *British Homeopathic Journal* **85**, 15-21.

Guillemain, J. et al. (1987) Pharmacologie de l'infinitésimal. Application aux dilutions homéopathiques. *Homéopathie* **4**, 35.

Harish, G. and Kretchmer, M. (1988) Smallest zinc quantities affect histamine release from peritoneal mast cells in rats. *Experientia* **44**, 761.

Homint R&D Newsletters: BOL 1998, Bukhsh 1999, Richter 1999, Knaff 2000, Heger 2001.

Jacobs, J. et al. (2000) Treatment of acute childhood diarrhoea with homeopathic medicine. *Paediatrics* **93**, 719.

Kaptchuk, T.J. (1997) Early use of blind assessment in a homeopathic scientific experiment. *British Homeopathic Journal* **86**.

Kayne, S. and Rafferty, A. (1994) The use of Arsenicum Album 30c to complement conventional treatment of neonatal diarrhoea in calves. *British Homeopathic Journal* **83**, 202.

Kleinen, J., Knipschild, P. and ter Riet, G. (1991) Clinical trials of homeopathy. *British Medical Journal* **302**, 316.

Lapp, C., Wurmser, L. and Ney, J. (1955) Mobilisation de l'arsenic fixe chez le cobaye sous l'influence des doses infinitésimales d'arséniate. *Thérapie* **10**, 625.

Linde, K. et al. (1997) Are the clinical effects of homeopathy placebo effects? A meta-analysis of placebo-controlled trials. *Lancet* **350**, 834.

Mahe, F. (1987) Evaluation of the effect of a collective homeopathic cure on morbidity and the butchering qualities in fattening calves. *International Journal of Veterinary Homeopathy* **2**, 13.

Nirmal, C. et al. (1987) Differentiation of potencies of Agaricus Muscarius by experimental catalepsy. *British Homeopathic Journal* **76**, July, 122–125.

Poitevin, B. (1995) Mechanism of action of homeopathic medicines. *British Homeopathic Journal* **38**, 32.

Reilly, D. et al. (1994) Is evidence for homeopathy reproducible? *Lancet* **344**, December.

Robinson, K. (1992) Hormesis. The Arndt-Schulz law rediscovered. *Homeopathic Links* 1/92.

Saxton J. (1991) Use of distemper nosode in disease control. *International Journal of Veterinary Homeopathy* **15**, 8.

Schiff, M. (1995) *The Memory of Water*. Wellingborough: Thorsons.

Searcy, R. and Guajardo, G. (1994) Papers on homeopathic research. *American Holistic Veterinary Medical Association Conference.*

Searcy, R., Reyes, O. and Guajardo, G. (1995) Control of subclinical bovine mastitis. *British Homeopathic Journal* **84**, 67.

Singh, P. and Chabra, H. (1993) Topological investigation of the water/ethanol system and its implications for the mode of action of homeopathic medicines. *British Homeopathic Journal* **82**, 164.

Towsey, M. and Hasan, M. (1995) Homeopathy. A biophysical point of view. *British Homeopathic Journal* 34, 218.

Vakil, A., Vakil, Y. and Nanabhai, A. (1989) Elevation of serum globulin levels in Chelidonium Majus provers. *British Homeopathic Journal* **78**, 97.

Van Galen, E. (1994) Homeopathy and morphic resonance. *British Homeopathic Journal* **83**, 63-67.

Williamson, A.V. et al. (1991) A study using Sepia 200c given prophylactically post partum to prevent anoestrus problems in the dairy cow. *British Homeopathic Journal* **80**, 149.

Williamson, A.V. et al. (1995) A trial of Sepia. *British Homeopathic Journal* **84**, 14-20.

Youbicier-Simo, B. et al. (1993) Effects of embryonic and in-ovo administration of highly diluted bursin on adrenocorticotropic and immune response of chickens. *International Journal of Immunotherapy* **9**, 169.

Chapter 3

The Remedies

There is often some confusion, when someone is introduced to homeopathy, over the use of the terms 'medicine' and 'remedy'. The conventional world, of course, always speaks of medicine, whilst in homeopathy we usually use the term remedy. This is not just to be different, but rather to emphasise the fact that the way homeopathy works is by encouraging the body to carry out its own 'remedial' work. The medicines of the conventional approach, in contrast, act in the main by concentrating merely on the removal of the presenting symptoms and the physiology and pathology associated with them.

Sources of the Remedies

Potentially a homeopathic remedy can be made from any substance, animal, vegetable, or mineral. Within this broad statement are a number of subdivisions, but in essence there is no limit to the healing potential within a substance that can be released by the homeopathic method. The sources may be classified as follows.

Animal. Either the whole animal is involved, as in the case of Apis Mellifica, where a complete honeybee is used, or else a product of a particular animal is taken as the starting point, for example, snake venom. There are two additional types of remedies which are of animal origin. *Sarcodes* are remedies made from healthy tissues, e.g. ovary. *Nosodes* are made from diseased tissues, discharges, and/or the causal agents of particular diseases.

Vegetable. Various individual parts or all of a plant may be utilised.

Mineral. These are obtained from a variety of sources as appropriate. The majority of these substances are used in their natural state, although man-made materials such as chemicals and conventional medicines may also be used. Some are also prepared from X-rays and more imponderable pure energy sources such as the sun and magnetic forces.

There are various homeopathic pharmacopoeias in use which provide the standards for the preparation of remedies. Although different countries may use slightly different references, there is broad agreement and increasing standardisation between them all and hence a common basis of standardised remedy manufacture is assured. There is control of the materials utilised as the sources of remedies, with detail of which part of a plant or animal is to be used, how a mineral is isolated and how it is to be prepared and stored.

Preparation of the Remedies

Many of the substances used to produce remedies are highly toxic in their material state. However, it must not be thought that the resulting homeopathic remedy is in any way similarly toxic. Indeed the most toxic substances, once in remedy form, are frequently among the most powerful healing agents. At the other end of the scale, substances that are conventionally thought of as inert can be converted into extremely useful medicines. The process of preparation of the homeopathic remedy is vital for this change. This process is called *potentisation* and, as the term implies, it is a means of making the original substance more potent as a healing agent. There are two essential stages in the process of potentisation – dilution and a procedure known as succussion.

Homeopathy is a therapy that works with the energy of the substances used rather than their physical form. The aim of potentisation is therefore to release the energy that is bound up in them and retain it in a usable form in the remedy. It is by this process that the healing potential of a substance is retained and enhanced, whilst the harmful aspects of the material form are removed.

The potency of the end product is expressed numerically in relation to the degree of dilution employed. Hahnemann found that the efficacy of the remedy increased with the degree of dilution, provided that the necessary succussion was also undertaken. There are three scales of dilution in use. Firstly, a decimal scale, based on a dilution of 1 in 10, is widely used in mainland Europe. This is denoted by the symbols 'D' or 'x'. While the decimal scale is also used to some extent in Britain, the majority of UK prescribing is based on the centesimal scale of 1 in 100, identified by the letter 'c'. This was the scale that Hahnemann originally produced, with the decimal scale being developed by others at a later date. In everyday usage the 'c' of centesimal is often omitted and just the number is quoted. There is also a third series of dilutions, known as the Q (quinquagintamillesimal) potencies. These are more commonly referred to as the LM (50 millesimal) potencies, as they are based on a dilution factor of 1:50,000. They represent Hahnemann's final development in relation to potency, as described in the 6th edition of the *Organon*. The major difference from the other potency scales lies in the method of dilution employed. Hahnemann came to think that the number of succussion stages that were employed in the preparation of a remedy had a major influence on the likelihood of severe reactions being produced in the patient. His aim was therefore to produce a gentler but still powerful remedy by obtaining a high degree of dilution without the corresponding number of succussion stages that would be necessary with the other scales. However, whichever scale is being used, the principle of potentisation by a combination of dilution and succussion is basically the same.

In order for dilution to be possible it is obviously necessary initially to produce a solution of the source material. The solvent used is an ethanol/water mixture and the initial solution is known as the *mother tincture*, denoted by the symbol φ. Some mother tinctures are also used as remedies for local application, or as organ-specific medicines, but their main purpose is as a stage in remedy creation.

Intrinsically soluble substances pose no problems, but for insoluble substances a process known as *trituration* must first be used. This involves the vigorous grinding of the substance with lactose powder in fixed proportion depending on the scale required. This is usually done as a three-stage process, and it is considered that this results in the energetic essence of the original substance being transferred to the lactose. The energised lactose can then be put into a solution and this point is equivalent to a 3c potency on the centesimal scale.

For the creation of the decimal and centesimal scales, one drop of mother tincture is then mixed with either 9 or 99 drops of solvent, as appropriate. This is then *succussed* (see opposite), and a 1D (or 1x) or 1c potency is thus created. One drop of this first potency is then mixed with a further 9 or 99 drops of solvent, succussion is repeated, and the second potency has been made. This process can be repeated as often as required. The diagram overleaf illustrates the process of remedy manufacture.

In the case of the LM potencies, the initial process is one of trituration, no matter what the source material. As mentioned above this process produces a 3c potency. This is then put into solution using 65mg of triturate and 500 drops (30ml) of a diluent comprising 100 drops of alcohol and 400 drops of water. This comprises what is called the *mother potency*. This is mixed with 100 drops of alcohol and succussed to create the LM1 potency. One drop of this is added to 100 drops of alcohol and succussed to form the LM2, and so on up to LM30. 100 succussions are used on each occasion to make the further potencies. As already mentioned, the name of the scale derives from the fact that the dilution at every stage is 1 in 50,000. LM30 is the maximum potency used, as Hahnemann considered that no body would be capable of reacting to a more powerful medicine than that.

It will be evident that all these methods will very rapidly produce extreme solutions. A 30c potency represents a dilution of 10 to the power of 60, and this is not considered to be an exceptionally high potency in practice. M (1000c) and 10M (10,000c) potencies are regularly employed, and even higher on occasion. Factors governing the selection of the appropriate potency are discussed in Chapter 8.

If homeopathic preparation were merely a matter of dilution then the critics would be correct (see Chapter 2), but this is where the all-important process of *succussion* becomes relevant.

Stated simply, succussion is nothing more than a vigorous shaking of the solution which takes place after each stage of dilution. However, its role in the creation of a remedy is vital. Homeopathic theory postulates that by means of this shaking the energy pattern of the original substance is transferred into the solvent. Water is crucial in this context – Victor Schauberger's work in the first half of the 20th century demonstrated the unique nature, not only of its physical character, but also of its dynamics, and the importance of vortex motion in its natural state (Alexandersson; Coates). It has also been shown that water can store information as energy patterns, provided that there is the requisite grouping of the molecules into clusters, and that the energy thus stored can affect its physical characteristics (Torres 2002).

Hahnemann was very clear as to the nature of the shaking required. It is not a violent indiscriminate shaking, but a strong rhythmic movement in the vertical plane. It is likely that this movement encourages a spiralling movement and the formation of vortices, which is necessary for the required molecular clusters to form. It has been demonstrated that in conditions of turbulence, vortices of varying sizes are found in a constant state of flux, and energy is known to move from the larger to the smaller. The exact nature of the shaking influences the energy input, and hence the resulting formation of vortices (Torres 2002). It is interesting to note that in the repetition of Benveniste's work discussed

The process of remedy manufacture

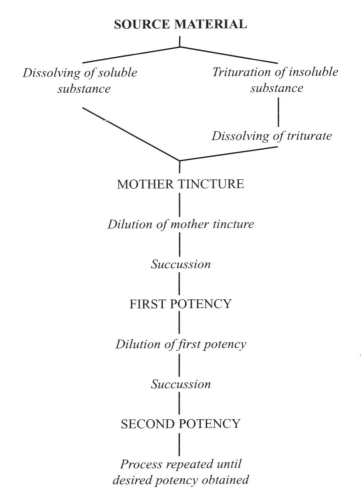

SOURCE MATERIAL

Dissolving of soluble substance | *Trituration of insoluble substance*

Dissolving of triturate

MOTHER TINCTURE

Dilution of mother tincture

Succussion

FIRST POTENCY

Dilution of first potency

Succussion

SECOND POTENCY

Process repeated until desired potency obtained

in Chapter 2, the method of preparation of the ultra-dilute solutions concentrated on the creation of vortices rather than using the traditional method of succussion.

Once the energy imprint is there it is retained, but the process of succussion must be repeated to ensure that it is passed on to the next dilution. When the concentration of the solute has fallen below Avogadro's number, of course, the distinction between solute and solvent has ceased to exist, as there are no longer any molecules of the original substance left. In fact, from the homeopathic point of view, it is irrelevant at any stage. From the beginning we are concerned purely with the energy that is inherent in the source material, and it is the process of succussion that primarily releases and magnifies that energy as a healing force.

As mentioned above, it is also thought that the process of trituration is more than just a thorough mixing with lactose powder and that the fine grinding involved is a vital part of the phenomenon of the transfer of the energy pattern. Although not scientifically proven, there must be some process of energy transfer during the grinding process, or the subsequent dilution and succussion stages would not result in a valid remedy, which they do.

Over the years many devices have been developed to produce the required high dilutions and aid in the mechanical production of the remedies. The details of most of these are not relevant to the present discussion, as they are not now widely used, but two methods are worthy of mention. The first is that of Korsakov, a Russian homeopath. Devised in 1829, the method allows for the more rapid manufacture of the higher potencies by utilising a single vial for the whole process rather than the separate vial at each stage that the Hahnemannian method requires. The first potency is prepared as for any centesimal process but then after each stage the vial is emptied, and the small quantity of liquid that is left on the glass inside the vial is taken as the starting point for the next dilution and succussion cycle. The exact dilution obtained by this process may thus be slightly different to that achieved by the original Hahnemannian method, and remedies produced by this method are designated by the letter 'K', e.g. 200K. Remedies produced by the original Hahnemannian method are sometimes denoted by adding the letter 'H' to the potency, e.g. 6DH or 30cH. Unless otherwise stated, the Hahnemannian method is presumed. Korsakov's method is still in use, although it is banned in France. This is linked more to restrictions over the use of high potencies generally that were introduced there in 1965 rather than to any deficiencies of the method.

The second variant is the process developed by Fincke in 1869 and known as *fluxion*. It too is a single vial method, and the potentising effect is obtained by the turbulence of water injected into the vial. It is generally considered to be not as reliable as the other methods, although a continuous fluxion apparatus was produced by Skinner, a Scottish physician (1825–1906), and this is still in occasional use.

In addition to the production of potencies as described above there is a technique known as *plussing*. This is not a means of bulk manufacture of a remedy, but is a method of slightly increasing the potency of each individual dose in a course of treatment. According to Hahnemann this slight adjustment of the potency on each occasion enhances the efficacy of the remedy and gives a gentle increase of the stimulant curative effect. The procedure, which is carried out by the owner or patient, has several variations, but essentially consists of dissolving the initial dose of the remedy in water and taking/administering it. The small quantity of fluid left in the glass is then used as the basis of the next dose, further water is added and stirred, and the process repeated for each administration. Although there are certain broad similarities with the Korsakov method of preparation, there is less accurate dilution, and less succussion, which results in only a slight increase in the potency. An alternative method which is used in acute cases is to dissolve the remedy in water and to succuss the whole between each administration. It is also a technique that is commonly employed during the administration of the LM potencies.

The Remedy Picture

In Chapter 1 it was stated that the principle 'let likes be treated by likes' is at the heart of homeopathy. In order to apply this, it is first necessary to know what the effect of a particular substance will be *on healthy individuals,* as the symptom picture that it is required to match will have been produced by the action of a disease agent on a healthy individual. Once this has been established, then the picture of the symptoms produced by the remedy can be matched to a disease picture presented by an animal. This knowledge, the 'remedy picture' as it is called, is obtained essentially from three sources.

The first of these is a **proving**. The term *homeopathic pathogenetic trial* is now being used increasingly to describe the process. In this the substance being investigated is administered to healthy volunteers, and the symptoms thus produced are noted. Hahnemann provided detailed instructions about how provings should be conducted, and he and his immediate followers 'proved' many of the major remedies that we use today. There has been a steady stream of work produced since by many researchers, both on new remedies and looking again at the older ones. Modern techniques involving control groups, randomisation and blinding have also been employed. Although doubts have been cast on the validity of much of the original work, these newer approaches have served largely to re-emphasise the basic accuracy of the original observations, even though some of the detail has been amended. Provings are carried out on humans, and thus the question of their accuracy in relation to animals arises. However, experience indicates that, with few exceptions, the results are readily transferable to animals and such experimental work as has been done would also support this (Chapter 13).

Toxicology is a further source of valuable information, with reports from cases of accidental poisoning providing additional data. Many conventional drugs produce a range of side effects, and although these are not strictly speaking poisonings, their effects can on occasions give a guide to their possible use as homeopathic remedies. Thus one of the hazards of the long-term use of potassium bromide in the treatment of epilepsy is the development of a skin reaction. In its homeopathic form, the remedy Kali Bromatum is used, where appropriate, to treat skin conditions due to other causes.

Clinical experience provides much knowledge of the remedies. One of the features of homeopathy is that effects and benefits may be seen in areas not being directly addressed in the presenting complaint. Thus successful treatment for a presenting reproductive problem may result in an improvement in the patient's arthritis, and this can lead to the future use of that remedy for treatment of a presenting arthritis.

Information yielded by the use of modern diagnostic techniques such as X-rays and blood tests is also relevant. Clinical experience also helps to confirm information from other sources, and also builds up knowledge of which types of patient respond best to particular remedies.

Experience of the use of a substance in a different therapeutic system, for example herbalism, may help our understanding. However, this cannot be relied on too much, as the sphere of action of a potentised substance may be very different to that of the crude substance from which it is derived.

In addition, much knowledge and understanding may be obtained by looking at an individual remedy as part of a group sharing certain characteristics or progressions. Thus considerations of the kingdom from which the remedy originates, or its position within the periodic table (as developed by Jan Scholten), or the common features of the plant or animal group from which it derives, can help to broaden and deepen the remedy picture. From such sources arises the concept of the *essence* of a remedy, which concentrates on the underlying characteristic themes of the group and patterns of behaviour that are exhibited, rather than on the detail of signs and symptoms that are the nuts and bolts of the materia medica.

The remedy pictures thus defined can initially appear daunting and at times contradictory. There is first of all a big difference between the amount of information provided about individual remedies. One reason for this is that some remedies have not been thoroughly proved and the information provided is derived mainly from clinical experience, which often concentrates on particular systems and conditions of the body. At the other end of the scale are remedies with extensive provings and of which there is much clinical experience. These are often what are known as *polychrests* – remedies that have such a wide range of action, incorporating all levels and systems of the body, that the clinical applications are widespread. These are the remedies that will be used daily in practice for a whole range of different conventionally named conditions.

Apparent contradictions will be found in the materia medica of these remedies, with both constipation and diarrhoea, dry and moist cough and so on being listed. It must be realised that remedies can present several pictures depending on the stage of the disease process; all symptoms are part of the whole, and the apparent anomalies are a reflection of this. The essence of the remedy will run through the whole picture. It must also be borne in mind that not every symptom of the remedy needs to be present in the patient before a successful prescription can be made.

One aspect of clinical experience that is also found is indications of relationships between remedies, with terms such as 'complementary', 'incompatible', 'follows well', 'antidotes', etc. These can give useful information in chronic prescribing as a means of remedy selection for the second or subsequent prescription. However, it must always be remembered that these guides only apply *after the first remedy has had an effect,* and the symptom picture has changed in some way.

Finally there is the concept of acute/chronic remedies. This is a special type of relationship that refers to the use of the connected remedies in particular circumstances. For example, Bryonia is said to be the 'acute' of Natrum Muriaticum. This implies that if a patient basically corresponds to the Natrum Muriaticum picture as far as chronic prescribing is concerned (see Chapter 9), then acute conditions in that patient will respond well to Bryonia. The relationship can be equally expressed as Natrum Muriaticum being the chronic of Bryonia, and in patients that have responded well to Bryonia for acute conditions, clinical experience teaches that chronic conditions are likely to respond to Natrum Muriaticum.

Storage and Dispensing of Remedies

As homeopathic remedies are essentially energetic in nature, various factors are important in relation to their storage and dispensing, which do not apply to the same extent to conventional drugs. However, any detrimental effects will only result in a loss of efficacy rather than inducing any untoward reactions in the patient. As with conventional medication, they should be kept in a dry environment. A moderate temperature range is also advisable. Opinions differ as to the exact effect of heat, with some authorities maintaining that there is no appreciable detrimental effect until temperatures reach around 150°F (65°C); on the other hand there is some evidence to suggest that 120°F (49°C) can be detrimental. Prolonged exposure will increase any detrimental effect. It is thus best to err on the side of caution and continuous exposure to elevated temperatures should be avoided. At the other extreme, although the temperatures produced by refrigeration will not necessarily harm them, it is not required for storage and the electromagnetic fields created by the refrigeration process are potentially harmful. Freezing of remedies should also be avoided. Exposure to a magnetic field of 50 Hz for 15 minutes has been shown to destroy the activity of remedies (Benveniste 1994). The temperature range for storage should be between 41°F (5°C) and 100°F (37.5°C). The effects of light, handling, strong smells and electrical emanations are the most significant.

Homeopathic remedies are particularly sensitive to light, so they should always be stored and dispensed in dark containers. Although plastic is acceptable for dispensing, long-term storage should always be in darkened glass. Even with suitable containers, storage in cupboards or drawers is preferable to that on shelves.

Handling should be avoided if possible and always kept to a minimum, as the energy of the handler will influence the remedy.

Strong-smelling substances can have a detrimental effect on the remedies. Thus exposure to garlic, camphor, peppermint and volatile substances in general must be avoided.

Microwaves, computers and other sources of energy waves are likely to be harmful to remedies, and close contact should be avoided.

The process of remedy preparation described above results in a liquid remedy of a given potency. This is then converted into the form required for administration.

Oral forms of remedies are available as tablets, pillules, granules or powder. The common base here is lactose powder that has been impregnated with the remedy. Sucrose or starch are also occasionally used. The only difference is one of size, with pillules being between tablets and granules. The potentised remedy in liquid form can also be used as drops for oral administration.

The most common and best route of administration is via a mucous surface. This is usually the mouth, but any other may be used. The mucosa of the vulval/vaginal region may be utilised by spraying a liquid form of the remedy directly onto the surface. Sprays can similarly be employed utilising the nasal passages. These latter two are of particular use where groups of farm animals require medication.

Injections are also a possibility, but their use is mainly confined to farm work. Their use is partly for convenience and partly to ensure that each animal in a group receives an adequate dose. Theoretically there are also issues of contamination associated with bulk medication of food or water and injections will avoid these, but in practice there does not appear to be any great advantage from injections in this connection.

In homeopathy the dose of a remedy that is employed is not directly related to the body weight of the patient (see Chapter 8); no matter what the physical size of the dose given at any one time, the body treats it as just one dose. This means that the dose administered at one time is usually only one tablet or pillule, or a 1gm pack of powder. Two or three drops of a liquid preparation are sufficient. Remedies given orally also act more effectively if they are absorbed through the mucosa of the mouth rather than being swallowed.

The usual instruction given to humans for taking remedies is to suck the tablet under the tongue until it dissolves. The mouth should also be clear of food or drink. Many practitioners insist on a period of abstention for at least half an hour either side of taking the remedy and also put bans on the consumption of tea, coffee, alcohol, etc. while using homeopathic medication.

For an animal the instruction to suck the remedy under the tongue is impractical, and many of the dietary considerations are not relevant here. But the principles behind the instructions are applicable to animals and can and should be followed. The mouth should be as clean as possible and strong-smelling substances should be avoided. For instance, peppermints given as a treat to a horse following dosage will interfere with the action of the remedy. On the other hand, garlic administered in a capsule that goes directly into the stomach will not interfere. In the larger companion animals, including horses, a clean mouth can be achieved by ensuring that feeding times avoid the times of remedy administration.

The sprinkling of a powder or crushed tablet into the mouth simulates as far as possible the sucking under the tongue. It is also possible to obtain tablets where the base will dissolve extremely quickly, and these can have many advantages in animals. In either case the saliva will quickly dissolve the lactose, thus aiding absorption through the mucosa. The fact that body weight is not a factor means that any slight loss from the mouth is immaterial. As in many animals the difficulty of tablet administration is getting them to swallow, rather than getting anything into the mouth, it will be seen that the homeopathic requirements in fact make dosage easier in many cases.

In the case of animals where handling of individuals is either difficult, dangerous or impractical, some compromise with the ideal method is unavoidable. If it is felt necessary to use food to disguise the medication, the mouth should be otherwise clean, and the 'bait' should be of a bland nature. Fruit with its high fluid content can be utilised, as the remedy will dissolve in the fluid and hence be easily absorbed. The remedy should not be mixed thoroughly into the food in an attempt to disguise it but should be left on the surface to ensure that it, rather than the food, is the first thing that comes into contact with the membranes. The drinking water can be a useful vehicle. If this method is used, it is important to ensure that all available sources of water are medicated. This is the most useful method with caged pets and is often the most practical way in herd or flock situations. The aim is to introduce the energy of the remedy into the water, and for this purpose dosage size is not as critical as it is in the conventional field. As a guide, a dosage of 1 ml per gallon (0.25 ml per litre) is sufficient.

The compromises that have on occasion to be made in the method of administration of a remedy will inevitably have some effect on its efficacy. For example, one of the most serious detrimental influences is that of light, and there is also the question of the irregularity of dosage to be considered when the drinking water is used as the vehicle. Although there will be occasions where the failure of a remedy to act is due to its method of administration, in most cases it appears that there may be a reduction in efficacy rather than a complete loss. There are implications for potency selection, duration of treatment, and interpretation of results in these cases but these can be accommodated. The important thing is to get the remedy into the patient(s) by some means. See Chapter 8 for a more detailed consideration of dosages.

References

Alexandersson, O. (1982) Living Water. *Viktor Schauberger and the Secrets of Natural Energy*. Bath: Gateway Books.

Benveniste, J. (1994) Further biological effects induced by ultra high dilutions. Inhibition by a magnetic field. In: Endler, P.C. and Schulte, J. (eds) *Ultra high dilution*. Dordrecht: Kluwer Academic Publishers.

Choudhary, H. (1990) *50-millesimal potency in theory and practice*. New Delhi: B. Jain Publishers.

Coats, C. (1996) *Living energies. Viktor Schauberger's Work Explained*. Bath: Gateway Books.

Dantas, F. (1996) A critique of provings. *British Homeopathic Journal* **85**, 2.

Torres, J-L. (2002) On the physical basis of succussion. *Homeopathy* **91**, 221-224.

Chapter 4

The Disease:
General Considerations

The Vital Force

Hahnemann's experiences with homeopathy inevitably led him to question the dynamics of the process of disease in an organism, and at length he developed a paradigm to explain his observations. He postulated that health and disease depend on the balance of what he termed the 'dynamis', an energetic manifestation that exerts a fundamental control over every aspect of the organism, keeping it in harmony. A morbific agent dynamically 'mistunes' the dynamis, and the expression of this mistunement is the production of symptoms. This concept of the 'dynamis' has been variously described as the 'vital energy' or 'vital force', and it is the latter term which has perhaps the most common usage.

The difference between this and the orthodox view is that in homeopathy the 'dis-ease' itself is considered to be the mistunement of the vital force, rather than the symptoms thereby produced. Naming the disease by labelling the symptoms is therefore of little advantage in understanding the process which is occurring. Similarly, any attempt to treat the disease must affect the vital force; once harmony in the vital force is restored the evidence of disease, in the form of the symptom complex, will disappear. This rebalancing of the vital force may be effected by the use of the appropriate homeopathic remedy.

In understanding this view of disease it is of paramount importance to understand what it is in a patient which needs to be cured. From the foregoing it will be apparent that it is the mistunement, or imbalance, in the vital force which must be returned to normal to effect a cure. Orthodox treatment with antipathic or allopathic drugs simply removes the symptoms, without having the necessary effect on the vital force. This is at least unproductive and indeed may be counterproductive. This is further explored in Chapter 5.

Challenging the Vital Force

As the vital force is a dynamic mechanism, it follows that any dynamic force may unbalance it. Thus mental and emotional shock, physical shocks and environmental effects can all unbalance the vital force, leading to symptoms of disease. Loss of a human or animal companion, or jealousy towards a new member of the family, can be potent initiators of disease, and the imbalance in the vital force so caused may then lead to physical symptoms. Similarly, a physical onslaught such as exposure to cold wind may so derange the vital force that symptoms of upper respiratory disease develop. Infectious diseases also affect the vital force, but it is essential in understanding the homeopathic concept of disease to realise that infectious agents such as distemper or feline calici virus exert their pathogenic effect by causing an imbalance in the vital force, which in turn reacts to produce the symptoms of disease. Each organism is governed by a unique and individual vital force; the consequence of this individuality is that the reaction of any one organism to a deranging force may well be different from that of another organism to the same force. This can be observed in the various manifestations of such a disease as canine parvovirus in any group of individuals. As a corollary to this, from a therapeutic point of view, two patients suffering from the same conventionally-named disease may, as stated earlier, need different homeopathic remedies.

From an orthodox viewpoint it is useful to consider what mechanisms are involved in the genesis of disease, and the immune system is perhaps the area to which one immediately turns. Certainly the major part of the practice of veterinary medicine is concerned with derangements of the immune system, either with acute or chronic infectious diseases or allergic phenomena such as atopy. An increasing number of autoimmune diseases have been identified, and even some of the endocrine diseases such as hypothyroidism are now being found to have an autoimmune basis (Dodds 1997). However, it is too simplistic to equate the immune system with Hahnemann's vital force, and to do so would relegate the concept from what is essentially an energetic one to the material. Similarly this would exclude an explanation for the emotional ('behavioural') diseases which are so commonly recognised among veterinary patients. One way of understanding the process is to consider the imbalance of the vital force as acting through the 'Psycho-Neuro-Endocrine-Immune axis' (PNEI). The 'central disturbance' to the PNEI axis results in the visible symptoms of disease which the practitioner observes. This may be the best way yet of conceptualising the vital force in an orthodox medical and veterinary framework and is indeed favoured by some of the world's leading homeopaths (for instance, Sankaran 1992).

Let us now consider what happens when the vital force is challenged. The vital force is unbalanced, setting in motion a process which results in symptoms being exhibited as an expression of this imbalance. It is in the interest of the vital force, as controller and maintainer of the organism, to limit these symptoms to less important, usually exterior, areas of the body. The skin or the mucous membranes of the nose are suitable levels at which to mount an initial defence. However, if the imbalance cannot be rectified, the vital force will become further weakened and more important organs such as liver or lungs may become affected. Eventually the most important organs such as the heart or brain are affected, and the patient may die.

Hering's Law

The inward march of disease has a corollary in the Law of Cure, attributed to Constantine Hering (1800–1880). This states that, in homeopathic terms, cure progresses:

- From interior to exterior
- From above downwards (in veterinary terms from head to tail and from body to extremities)
- From more important organs to less important organs

and that:

- Symptoms disappear in the reverse order of their appearance

In simple cases these are phenomena which can be readily observed in animals undergoing homeopathic treatment. Where the case has been complicated by the passage of time and by prolonged orthodox medical treatment, they may not always be seen so clearly. However, an understanding of Hering's Law is an essential step in understanding the concepts behind the homeopathic view of disease.

From the discussion so far, it should be apparent that disease in this context can no longer be named or described in simple terms. The imbalance in the vital force cannot be observed or labelled, but the evidence for its existence is present in the form of symptoms. In this context the word 'symptom' includes everything which has changed in the patient. In addition any disturbance in the PNEI axis will have effects on all its parts. It follows that in any case of disease, along with the physical symptoms there are changes in the mental demeanour and in the 'general' symptoms – the thirstlessness and languor of the cat with calicivirus are as much parts of the symptom complex as the sneezing and the ulcerations on the tongue. In homeopathic parlance this concept is described as the 'totality' of symptoms; in other words the homeopathic case consists not only of the symptoms for which the animal is presented, but of all the symptoms exhibited by that individual. Hence the totality of symptoms exhibited by a horse with colic is represented by irritability, restlessness and sweating, along with the gut pain itself.

Homeopathic medicine aims to redress the imbalance in the vital force, and so instigate a process which results in the elimination of the symptoms. This is in direct contrast to much of the orthodox medicine which is used in the veterinary field, designed as it is to directly oppose the symptoms themselves. In homeopathic terms, the use of anti-inflammatories, antidiarrhoeals, immunosuppressives such as cortico-steroids, and even antibiotics are seen as merely *suppressing* the symptoms, and not dealing with the imbalance in the vital force, the central disturbance of the PNEI axis.

As the homeopath sees it, the effect of this suppression is to drive the symptoms deeper into the organism. If the vital force is strong enough it will react by throwing up symptoms elsewhere, but on the same level; a skin lesion treated with corticosteroid cream may lead to otitis externa. If the vital force is not of sufficient strength, deeper organs will be affected, such as intestines or lungs. The effects of suppression are very real, and can be observed in any veterinary consulting room if sufficient time is taken to closely observe how a chronically ill patient has developed in its symptomatology. This is not to deny the obvious benefits which modern veterinary medicine can at times provide, but in the study of homeopathy it is essential to be aware of the consequences of suppressive medical treatment. Only when this is fully acknowledged can steps be taken to remedy its effects.

One Disease at a Time

If the expression of disease results from a mistunement or imbalance of the vital force, it follows that only one disease pattern can be present at one time. If the vital force is challenged with sufficient power as to cause further imbalance, but in a different way, a new set of symptoms will arise. When a new disease pattern occurs in this way, the original symptoms will be suspended. Once the new disease has run its course or been cured, the old symptoms will recur. This phenomenon can be recognised in practice where, for instance, a dog suffering from a chronic skin disease contracts acute gastroenteritis. The skin symptoms will often abate for the duration of the gastroenteritis, but on recovery from the latter, the pruritus returns.

It is important to remember that any imbalance in the vital force may produce symptoms which in a conventional sense might be termed separate diseases, such as pyoderma and colitis, but from a homeopathic view, if they coexist they are considered to be part of the same disease complex.

All the foregoing assumes that the new disease force is stronger than the original disease force. If the reverse is true, then the patient will be protected from the deranging effects of the new disease force by which it is challenged. Using the example of the chronically itchy dog, it follows that if the original disease is strong enough, in other words the disease is deeply enough entrenched, this patient will be less likely to suffer from the mild viral epidemic diarrhoea or kennel cough outbreaks to which other, 'healthier' dogs may be prone. Once again, observations in practice corroborate this. An interesting historical example is provided by medical reports of eighteenth century lunatic asylums where the inmates are reported to have been surprisingly free of other forms of disease, mental disease representing a deeper level of disease than those on the physical plane and therefore, by definition, 'stronger'.

In Paragraph 40 of the *Organon*, however, Hahnemann does concede that in the rare occasions where two diseases of similar strength but of sufficient dissimilarity occur, they can combine to form a complicated disease. A patient suffering from chronic colitis could therefore suffer from a corneal ulcer without affecting the enteric symptoms.

From the above comes the concept that a patient may suffer from 'layers' of disease – weaker diseases having been suppressed by stronger ones. As homeopathic treatment resolves the presenting symptom complex, those symptoms associated with the previous disease are exhibited. This 'recrudescence phenomenon', as it is known, can often be witnessed in an animal treated successfully with homeopathy. Sometimes the emergent symptom complex resolves spontaneously, at other times another homeopathic remedy is necessary, based on the new symptoms. There is further discussion of this in Chapter 7.

Where disease processes are similar, the stronger one annihilates the weaker, and the action of a homeopathic remedy may be considered to be that of a similar, but stronger, disease. The effect of the remedy is to dislodge the effect of the disease on the vital force, allowing the latter to return to harmony. The homeopathic remedy, being dynamic in nature, ceases to exist after it has exerted its effect.

Primary and Secondary Actions

Hahnemann spent much of his life observing the effects of medicines, both orthodox and homeopathic, on the human organism, and he concluded that the effects of medicines comprised an action and a re-action. The initial action of the medicine on the organism is strong enough to exert a deranging force and produce symptoms itself. This is termed the **primary action** of the remedy, and while it is primarily due to the action of the remedy itself, the vital force inevitably also plays a part, albeit small. In the main the role of the vital force in the primary action is a passive one. Very rapidly, however, it reacts against the effects of the medicine. This is the **secondary action** (or **counteraction**) and where such an effect exists in nature, is exactly opposite to the primary action. One example cited by Hahnemann is that of coffee, used as a stimulant: once the primary, stimulatory, effect has worn off, the patient feels even more drowsy than before, due to the secondary reaction of the vital force counteracting the effect of the drug. The drowsiness may last for some considerable time and the only way to overcome it is to take an even larger dose of coffee. Another example is the longstanding constipation which may follow the more acute effects of a laxative.

These effects explain the phenomenon, so frequently encountered in veterinary practice, whereby ever-increasing doses of conventional medicines are necessary to maintain their therapeutic effects. With homeopathic medicines, the primary and secondary actions are usually so mild as to largely go unnoticed, and the only effect which is observed is the gentle return to normal engendered by a vital force returned to harmony. However, in sensitive patients the primary action may be observed in the form of a temporary worsening of symptoms following the administration of the remedy, the so-called 'homeopathic aggravation'. (This is dealt with more fully in Chapter 8.) The reaction here may be termed a curative secondary action, to distinguish it from the secondary counteraction encountered with material doses of medicines.

Secondary counteraction is seen when the contrasting phenomena are seen in nature as part of the normal processes of physiological balance, e.g. diarrhoea and constipation. Secondary curative action occurs when the balance has been upset and requires re-establishment, as in disease. The homeopathic concept of disease and cure, then, is one of a dynamic process which involves the imbalance of the controlling vital force; the consequence being that symptoms appear in the organism to manifest the imbalance. A correctly prescribed homeopathic remedy represents a similar dynamic agent which restores the vital force to harmony. This instigates a restorative process, the result of which is the removal of the symptom complex. The observation that the symptoms have been completely removed assures the practitioner that the patient has undergone cure.

References

Dodds, J. (1997) Autoimmune thyroiditis and polyglandular auto-immunity of purebred dogs. *Canine Practice* **22**(1), 18-19.

Sankaran, R. (1999) *The Spirit of Homeopathy* (3rd edn). Mumbai, India: Homeopathic Medical Publishers.

Chapter 5

The Disease:
Manifestations of Disease

The Nature of Disease

Disease may be classified into two main categories. Firstly there is the acute, where the illness comes on quickly and runs its course, resulting, in most cases, in either recovery or death over a relatively short period of time. In some situations it is possible for a state of chronic disease to become established, due to such factors as an over-concentration on the removal of particular symptoms rather than viewing and treating the disease as a whole.

Secondly, there is chronic disease. From the conventional point of view the major implication is that a condition has been present for a considerable period of time. There is usually also the perception that the condition is incurable, and hence that palliation is the best that can be achieved. It is important at all times to distinguish between cure and the relief of symptoms.

The long-term use of agents such as anti-inflammatory drugs in these situations can lead to confusion between genuine cure and the relief of the symptoms, which is not of itself necessarily curative.

Homeopathically there is a different perception of chronic disease. Although time is certainly a factor, more important is the concept of the process as a profound imbalance in the body's dynamics which manifests itself clinically in more than one system, either concurrently or at different times.

Conventionally a patient would therefore be regarded as suffering with arthritis as one condition, periodic colitis as another, and maybe eczema as a third. Each presenting complaint is put in a separate compartment and each perceived condition is treated separately. In contrast, homeopathy views all the signs and symptoms as being indications of one underlying 'dis-ease', and seeks to treat the underlying imbalance by viewing the patient as a whole. What is also seen on occasion is the acute flare-up of an aspect of an underlying chronic disease. It is important to differentiate such a case from a true acute disease, and although it may be necessary in the short term to treat it in the same way as a genuine acute disease, its connection to the ongoing deep-seated condition must not be forgotten. In one sense the homeopathic approach to the treatment of disease is the same, irrespective of whether one is dealing with an acute or chronic condition. The aim is to find the remedy that is the *simillimum* – that is, the one that most closely matches the total symptoms of the patient. However, in an acute illness, the emphasis is usually on the more local signs.

That is not to say that the general and mental symptoms are not of use, and it can be particularly important to note any changes from normal that occur in these during illness. But, by the very nature of an acute condition, the picture that is presented is often limited in its range, and time is often of the essence. The prescription is thus often based mainly on the major features of the symptomatology that mirror major features of the remedy. Acute disease can potentially affect any animal, and this implies that there will be a wide range of age and vitality among the patients. Those that are essentially young and fit will have a strong vital force, which will be able to mount a strong response to the challenge, and this will result in the production of many clear-cut symptoms. Weaker animals with a lower vital force will correspondingly present a less well defined disease picture.

By contrast, in chronic disease conditions the vital force will inevitably have been weakened to some degree by the disease process, and although the range of signs and symptoms that are available to guide the choice of remedy may involve a greater number of body systems, there may not be such a clear-cut picture as in the acute disease situation.

The treatment of the two types of disease also involves different considerations of potency and frequency of administration, and these are discussed in Chapter 8; for the moment it is enough to appreciate the exact approach to be followed when attempting to cure the patient.

It has been said that homeopathy never cured anything – all it does is to help the body to cure itself. This is one way of summarising the homeopathic approach, where the signs and symptoms on which remedy selection is based are the result of the body's attempt to restore the internal balance that is recognised as health. The symptoms that are produced in this process are the result of the vital force acting through the body's systems, and by using these as the guide to remedy selection the systems are being stimulated by the treatment in just those areas that are most appropriate to produce a cure. The body will attempt to produce its cure in accordance with Hering's Law (Chapter 4), and by following at all times the clues that the body gives it ensures that the greatest of all medical maxims – to *assist nature* – is followed.

The appearance of pyrexia, inflammation, and the other signs of the body's reaction are regarded by the conventional world firstly as a means of diagnosis, and secondly as symptoms to be removed *as a means of* achieving a cure. Homeopathically they are the guides to the remedy and are removed *as a result of* achieving a cure.

The body's reactions to challenge are aimed solely at restoring health, and they always have a positive aim in that regard: for instance, an elevated body temperature increases the efficacy of phagocytosis, and its appearance in the symptom picture is an indication of the body's efforts to restore health. While too high a fever can in certain circumstances be detrimental, and measures must be taken to counteract it, in general terms the artificial suppression of pyrexia can in fact hinder recovery.

As already mentioned in Chapter 4, Hering's Law implies that the reactions of the body are designed to throw any disease process outwards, away from the vital organs, and in this context vital means in relation to survival. The ultimate expression of this is seen when treatment of a disease initially affecting the vital organs leads to the involvement of the skin, which is, from the survival point of view, the least important organ of all. This same outward movement of the disease process may of course also be seen during any successful defence by the body to challenge, irrespective of any treatment. In either case this will result in either a definite physical lesion, or a purely functional upset such as pruritis, with a corresponding improvement in the deeper systems that were affected. Either way it is a manifestation of the Law of Cure in action.

Nature always aims to provide an outlet for the disease process at as superficial a level as possible, but if this aim is blocked the disease will be expressed at a deeper and potentially more serious level. Any interference with the natural process of exteriorisation will have the effect of halting the curative efforts of the body, with the result that the disease picture is forced to find expression in other directions, which will inevitably be in the deeper and more important organs.

Thus any treatment which has the aim of removing a symptom without due regard as to why that symptom is present, and without regard to the totality of the picture, is liable to result in a *suppression* of the natural curative process. If these treatments are persevered with in a case of acute disease, the result may be the creation of a state of chronic disease. Similarly, the use of suppressive treatments in established chronic cases will then cause a further deepening of the disease process.

It must be remembered that suppression can occur, not only from the use of conventional medications, but also via the use of many of the 'natural' therapies. Homeopathy itself can be used in a way that blocks the natural curative response if the remedy is selected on a very narrow range of symptoms that reflect the disease as it affects only one system or function, but which do not represent the totality of the disease. The relief of the symptoms may thus be only palliative, and continued use of the remedy in this way can lead on to a true suppression and deepening of the disease. Care must also be taken to avoid suppression when combining the use of different therapies in a case.

Suppression can also occur in healthy animals when medicinal agents or other procedures are used to interfere with and control normal body functions. This practice is mainly encountered in the reproductive field although there are other areas of potential harm. The use of chemicals or surgery to control any normal physiological function is itself a form of suppression. Even artificial stimulation of systems can lead to upsets in the natural balance, and the use of prostaglandins etc. to increase and regulate reproductive activity can produce problems in the long term. It may be that in some cases, such as surgical neutering, there are valid reasons for such procedures; but if they are employed consideration should always be given to the effect that they will have on the patient's ability to function normally in response to disease.

Whilst most of the clinical problems that are met with in practice as a result of these procedures will be seen in the companion animals, this does not mean that the farmed species do not suffer from the same abuses. The only difference is that commercial considerations usually lead to a failure to consider the importance of the clinical effects from the point of view of the individual animal. Indeed, such is the lesser importance of the individual animal in the farm situation that animals are either routinely disposed of before clinical conditions manifest themselves, or else affected animals are culled once symptoms have appeared.

Attitudes to Disease

The difference between the concepts of chronic disease in the conventional and the homeopathic disciplines has already been mentioned. One of the basic tenets of conventional medicine is the reductionist approach, which consequently tends to concentrate on pathology. Because this is such a major part of conventional thinking, it means that sight is easily lost of the whole disease process as understood by homeopathy, and conventionally there is no appreciation of the true relationship between function and pathology. This has two consequences. The first is the confusion that is found at times between the relief of symptoms and a cure, which leads to palliation. The second is that the relief of symptoms is often considered by the conventional world to be a prerequisite of a curative process.

Once disease is viewed in that light, the removal of the symptoms of disease becomes the aim of treatment, resulting in the development of drugs to meet this perceived need. Hence there are the anti-inflammatory drugs, the antipyretics and to some extent the antibiotics. Antibiotics, of course, do have valuable uses that are consistent with the requirement of all valid treatments to assist nature. They are, however, essentially short-term agents when used correctly, and their long-term use – for example where there is secondary infection in chronic skin conditions – is aimed solely at controlling what is perceived as the disease. In these cases the use of antibiotics, especially when linked with anti-inflammatories, has the effect of blocking the working-through of the full curative process. Such blocking, as explained above, has the effect of driving the disease process inwards towards the vital organs. Since such 'skin cases' are in fact part of a wider chronic disease picture in the body, the overall result is a worsening of the total disease.

The same attitude to symptoms can also contribute to the conversion of an acute disease into a chronic one. As discussed in Chapter 4, the development of symptoms through the action of the vital force is the basis of the body's response to, and attempt to deal with, the challenge that faces it. In an acute infectious condition, for example, part of that reaction may be an elevation of the body temperature, which in its wake may bring aching muscles and a headache. (There is no reason to suppose that these symptoms are not present in animals just as much as in humans.) If treatment is aimed primarily at the removal of these symptoms, it may well involve the artificial reduction of the (desirable) pyrexia, with the consequence that the body's ability to meet its challenge is compromised. This is just as much a suppression of the curative process as any that has been discussed and, as indicated above, will result in the inward movement of the disease process. Hence overdue concern for the immediate comfort of the patient may well be counterproductive as far as a genuine and complete cure is concerned.

At the other end of the scale, of course, it is essential to avoid unnecessary suffering, and this is without doubt a major consideration at all times. However, there is a world of difference between *necessary discomfort* and *unnecessary suffering,* and to avoid the former by producing a short-term palliation at the expense of establishing a chronic disease that will cause further long-term ill-health is not in the best interests of the patient. Nature's priority is not that an individual will never become ill, but that they are able to recover and be healthy. It is important to realise that any obstruction of the natural unfolding of the curative process may lead to problems in the future.

This is one area where homeopathy has many advantages. Because correctly selected remedies encourage the natural processes of the body to work through more quickly, their use in acute conditions can avoid the creation of chronic problems, whilst at the same time bringing the required relief to the patient by way of a genuine cure rather than by a suppression of temporarily uncomfortable symptoms. Nor need this be a long process. In Paragraph 2 of the *Organon,* Hahnemann states that 'The highest ideal of cure is the rapid, gentle and permanent restoration of health', and in acute disease this is usually attainable.

A rapid cure is not so easily attained in cases of chronic disease, and here the timescale is often linked to the amount of suppressive treatment that the patient has received. A rule of thumb sometimes quoted among homeopaths is that one month of homeopathic treatment is required for each year of conventional treatment that has been received. Whilst this is not a hard and fast rule, and should not be quoted as such, it nevertheless gives a flavour of the problems that can be encountered.

Another feature of the successful homeopathic treatment of a chronic condition is that the process may be accompanied by the reappearance of old symptoms (Hering's Law, page 43). These may involve a degree of discomfort and/or inconvenience, and in such cases it is important to remember the requirement not to halt the curative process by overconcentration on the temporary relief of what will normally be transient phenomena.

Hahnemann's Concept of Chronic Disease

Although Hahnemann and his followers were able to produce many successful cures by following the simillimum principle, they also had many cases where either apparently well-indicated remedies failed to produce the expected result, or where the initial improvement was not maintained. More than that, the disease would often re-appear in a stronger form, or a new set of symptoms would appear after the apparent resolution of the condition. At first there was some thought that this might be happening solely because of the small number of remedies that had been adequately proved, but as more remedies became available the situation did not improve and it was clear that there were other factors involved. Hahnemann's observation that many of the conditions returned in a modified form, with some new symptoms, led him to the view that in these cases he was not dealing with a well defined and easily classified disease, but was in fact only seeing one aspect of a deep-seated underlying condition. From this start, after some twelve years of investigations, he produced his *Miasmatic Theory of Chronic Disease,* which is a model that accounts for the observed phenomena of clinical practice.

This theory, which is discussed in greater detail in Chapter 11, postulated that all chronic disease is the result of one or more of three basic influences acting abnormally on the vital force. Hahnemann called these influences *psora, sycosis* and *syphilis.* His concept of them was initially explained in terms of the major clinical entities of his time, with *psora* equating to scabies, *sycosis* to gonorrhoea and *syphilis* to syphilis in its conventional form. As a result they are often thought of, even today, as some form of infectious agent, whereas his ideas were broader than that. He felt that the suppression of the normal body reactions to disease was the major factor, and that chronic disease was being created by a basic failure to understand the true nature of the body's healing process.

Hahnemann considered that the ancient physicians were in many cases attempting to treat disease correctly, but that their limited resources resulted in a suppression and consequently the establishment of chronic disease. However, he accused his orthodox contemporaries of more misdirected and deliberately harmful practices, and not surprisingly this did not endear him to them! His contention was that in all such cases the disease was being driven inwards rather than being brought out as nature intended, and that this was the vital difference between the two approaches.

This theory of miasms split the emerging homeopathic world. Some physicians abandoned homeopathy altogether, unable to accept where it was going. Others felt that while Hahnemann had been correct in his earlier concepts this was an idea too far, and continued to practice as they had been doing before, thereby getting some positive results but also many failures. A third group accepted the theory wholeheartedly and set about incorporating it in their work.

These early reactions have been perpetuated in the attitude to the theory among homeopaths over the years, and as a consequence there have been times when miasmatic theory has been largely ignored. Even Hering, one of Hahnemann's greatest followers and advocates, at one time doubted the validity or relevance of the theory, but later came to appreciate its value. His initial view was that it was irrelevant 'whether a physician [accepts] the theory, as long as he always selects the most similar medicine possible'. Today there are also some authorities who question its validity and relevance to prescribing.

There is no doubt that it is possible to practice homeopathy without following the precepts of miasmatic theory as a major prescribing tool, and many competent homeopaths do so. Proponents of the theory would consider that, although such people are not actively considering the miasmatic approach, nevertheless their prescribing methods do in fact take account of the miasmatic aspects of their cases. J.H. Allen, in his book on the miasms, advocates the theory as being 'the difference between intelligent warfare and fighting in the dark, as what we see from our patients is only about some small fragment of a deep-seated disease'.

The early idea that the problems and failures of treatment were the result of the limited range of remedies available to Hahnemann and his colleagues still has some credence today, with some authorities (e.g. Massimo Mangialavori) essentially holding that view, and considering that a greater understanding of the remedies and improved prescribing will overcome the problems. Against that it can be argued that the valuable new insights into remedies that are being introduced by workers such as Vithoulkas, Sankaran and Scholten, while dramatically changing prescribing methods, are having little significant effect on the successful treatment of chronic disease.

Modern insights into pathological processes and the developments in genetics are confirming the soundness of Hahnemann's basic understanding of the nature of chronic disease. Many of the conditions for which genetic aberrations are now being found can be equated with psora, and developments in asthma research are expressing the same view of the condition as miasmatic considerations lead to. Clinical experience is indicating that miasmatic influences are capable of being passed from generation to generation in ways other than those recognised by established Mendelian patterns Although there is still some disagreement over the detailed interpretation of his concepts, there is now an increasing acceptance of the usefulness of the theory's framework as a prescribing tool.

References

Allen, J.H. (1908) *The Chronic Miasms Psora and Pseudopsora.* Chicago.

Cole, J. and Dyson, R. (1997) *Classical Homeopathy Revisited.* West Wickham: Winter Press.

Chapter 6

Obtaining the Symptoms

Signs and Symptoms

These two terms mean slightly different things. Signs are essentially objective, whereas symptoms are more subjective on the part of the patient. There is often an overlap in the way the terms are used, with 'symptom' being used to include signs as well, but it is always helpful to bear the difference in mind. Broadly, conventional medicine is more concerned with signs rather than symptoms, while homeopathy concerns itself as much, if not more, with symptoms rather than signs. However, when using homeopathy on animals, many of the subjective elements of a case are unobtainable. Some inferences can validly be made, but there is inevitably a greater reliance on signs alone than is met with in human practice.

One great difference between the conventional and homeopathic approaches to disease, and therefore to case taking, is that whereas the conventional world concentrates on what is standard about a case, the homeopathic approach is to attempt to elicit and use those aspects that are peculiar to the individual. The whole object of case taking for the homeopath is to be able to make the subsequent prescription as individual to the patient as possible. Hence much that is valuable to the homeopath is dismissed as irrelevant by the conventional veterinary surgeon. The converse is not, however, true. The homeopathic veterinary surgeon will take account of the conventional diagnosis and those signs that led to it, but will give them a lower priority than their conventional colleague. From the homeopathic point of view, a sign or symptom will only become really valuable if an individual dimension can be given to it.

It will be realised from the above that many of the signs and symptoms used by conventional veterinary surgeons to reach a diagnosis are of limited value to the homeopathic prescriber. They are what are termed *common* symptoms – signs such as diarrhoea, conjunctivitis and so on that will be found in most cases of a particular disease.

Equally, signs which do not appear in a particular case of a disease, but which are present in the majority of cases, become significant. For example, increased thirst is a usual feature in a case of pyometra and is hence of little use in homeopathic prescribing; but in a case of pyometra with no increase in the thirst this fact can be of significance.

At the other end of the scale are the *strange, rare, and peculiar* symptoms (SRP). The term *peculiar, queer, rare, and strange* (PQRS) is sometimes used to denote the same symptoms. These are the features of an individual case or patient that are unique. The conventional world is very likely to ignore these, or downgrade their significance, as they do not fit into the standard framework that is the basis of that approach.

To a homeopathic prescriber, the less a symptom can be explained by the disease process the more significant it is. Hence these are among the most valuable of all. These two extremes of common and 'strange, rare and peculiar' symptoms, are the lower and upper points of a definite hierarchy of symptoms, which is used to grade the importance of the information obtained. Starting from the upper end this continues in the order of:

Strange, rare and peculiar symptoms

Hahnemann rated these as the most significant symptoms of all, as they represent the ultimate in individualisation. Paragraph 153 of the *Organon* states that 'these, above all, must correspond to very similar ones (symptoms) in the symptom set (remedy picture) of the medicine sought if it is to be the most fitting one for cure'. There may be occasions when the prescription will be decided by these symptoms.

Mental symptoms

These are concerned with temperament and personality. Fears and phobias, likes and dislikes at a mental level, anger, jealousy, excitability and sociability come into this group. The mental state in health is of as much interest as in disease, and any changes arising consequent upon the disease are of great significance. Within the mental symptoms those that can be linked to an aetiology – e.g. fright or grief – are also to be rated highly. This is referred to as 'causality' and represents the significant connection of events in the past to the current presenting picture.

General symptoms

Here the emphasis is on the physical characteristics of the patient, and the picture in both health and disease is important. The owner of an animal will usually preface the information with 'he/she', indicating that the observed phenomenon is a feature of the whole animal rather than any particular part of it. Reactions of the body to temperature, and desires or aversions to particular foods, are examples of such symptoms. Thus a desire for crisps in a dog could be due to a desire for salt, which could be used as a general symptom. However, other constituents in the product may be the attraction, and so it is necessary to be absolutely clear as to what the desire really is before it can be utilised. As with mental symptoms, any changes due to the illness are of most significance.

One general symptom used in homeopathy is that of laterality, and reference will be found to particular remedies being 'left' or 'right' sided. This means that in a particular individual there is a marked preference for one side or the other, and any conditions will tend to show symptoms on that side of the body. For example, conditions that require Phosphorus as a remedy will manifest symptoms primarily on the left side of the body. Even in health the Phosphorus type will prefer not to lie on the left side. However, this concept must not be pushed too far as an absolute. Conditions may start on a particular side, but as the disease progresses the other side may also become involved. Indeed, it is a feature of some remedies that symptoms appear first on one side then extend to the other.

Local symptoms

Sometimes called 'particular symptoms', these are concerned with the presenting complaint(s) and any associated pathology. To the conventionally trained practitioner these are usually the most important, and the patient or owner will also consider them so. Although they are of use in selecting the remedy, they are not as important in the homeopathic prescription as the others above.

Common symptoms

These are the least important from the homeopathic point of view, although the conventional diagnosis will usually be based on them. They are generally too vague to be of use in homeopathic remedy selection. If they can be personalised, however, they can become of use.

The exact nature of a diarrhoea, or the precise colour and volume of an ocular discharge, can make what started as a common symptom more valuable.

Modalities

A modality is not a symptom but rather a factor that changes the nature of a sign or symptom. Modalities are an important part of every remedy and disease picture and for this reason, when a symptom is elicited in a case, the practitioner should try to link it with a modality. For instance, it may be established that a particular animal has a tendency towards flatulence. Further questioning may establish the fact that this tendency is more marked after eating. 'Worse after eating' is therefore the modality of flatulence in this case.

A modality either ameliorates or aggravates the symptom. This is designated respectively by the symbols > (better for) and < (worse for). The modalities that are of most use in veterinary work are those regarding temperature, movement, eating, time, touch (pressure), and weather.

Modalities can occur at all levels, and the same factor may have different effects at different levels. A skin irritation may be aggravated by heat although the animal as a whole may prefer heat. The preference for heat is a general symptom in its own right, while the aggravation of the skin by heat is a modality of a local symptom. Equally, the animal as a whole may be upset by heat and the skin irritation increased. This is a modality of a general symptom.

Concomitant symptoms

Concomitant symptoms are symptoms that are present in the patient but which do not appear to have any direct connection with the presenting complaint. They are all classified into one of the groups discussed above, but the concept is important for the interpretation and analysis of a case. They can be in another area and sometimes at another level in the symptom picture, and the more unlikely the connection, the more valuable the symptom becomes.

They are often the sort of thing that the conventional approach, with its tendency to compartmentalise, regards as irrelevant, and are an aspect of the need in homeopathy to think laterally.

For example, a dog may present with repeated episodes of acute diarrhoea which are always accompanied by an intense irritation of the left ear. The involvement of the left ear is a concomitant symptom of the diarrhoea. In terms of homeopathy there is likely to be a connection via a remedy, whereas there is no conventional explanation as to why these two symptoms should appear together.

Complete symptoms

Complete symptoms are characterised by having the four components of location, aetiology, modality and sensation (or characteristic) associated with them. Sensation in veterinary work can be difficult to ascertain, but in general terms the more complete a symptom is, the more significant it becomes, and the more helpful it is in making a prescription.

Keynote symptoms

Strictly speaking these may be regarded as a feature of a remedy rather than of a patients, but it is convenient to include them at this point. A keynote is an unusually strong feature of a remedy and will be strongly emphasised in any description of that remedy. The feature of Bryonia of being worse for movement is an example. When this modality is seen in a case it is a strong indication for prescribing the remedy, although the final prescription will take other features into account.

Taking the Case

This is the key to successful homeopathic practice, as the ability to match symptoms to known remedy pictures lies at the heart of the method. The diverse nature of veterinary work involving companion, farm and other working animals leads to differences of case-taking technique, but the requirement of the simillimum applies to all. There are two basic parameters which must be borne in mind:

i) There is no such thing as irrelevant information

ii) No information is better than wrong information.

The term 'unprejudiced observer' is sometimes used to describe the ideal role of the clinician in case-taking. There is always the temptation to be guided by an owner towards what they consider the most important aspects of the condition. These are almost invariably the local signs and are often, as already discussed, the less important features from the homeopathic point of view. Some owners also have a tendency to rationalise the things that are happening in the case: these explanations must, however, be regarded with a degree of caution. Not only do they represent the very personal interpretation of the owner, but their relevance to the information required to make a prescription is usually limited. In veterinary work this tendency can be compounded by the assumption on the part of the practitioner that the mental and general symptoms are too difficult to obtain, and hence most prescribing must be at a local level. Although this may be true in some cases it must *not* be allowed to become a mind-set.

The obtaining of mental and general symptoms is not necessarily as difficult as it may appear to a beginner. As in the human field, the most successful prescribing is done when the higher levels of the mental and general symptoms are incorporated in the picture. The key to successful case-taking is good observation and good communication. It must always be remembered that there is a relationship between the owner and the animal that can yield useful information. The nature of this relationship can often be ascertained by observation, plus a degree of lateral thinking about what the owner actually says.

There is also, of course, the relationship between the veterinary surgeon and the owner to consider. Add in the relationship between the vet and the animal and the interaction of these three can make for some interesting times!

The acute case

This is met with in all types of practice, and commercial considerations will mean that much farm work falls into this category. As has been seen, an acute condition arises relatively quickly and presents a limited but usually fairly well defined range of signs.

The prescription is mainly based on these signs, which are then matched with the more major features of the remedy. They tend to be mainly local with some easily recognised general symptoms that represent the dominant physical characteristics of the patient. The mental symptoms are not used to the same extent in the acute situation as they are in the chronic. However, they must not be ignored and if present should be utilised, as strong mental symptoms can be of great help. What is particularly useful is any change in a mental or general symptom as a result of the illness. Some exploration into such aspects of the case other than the presenting physical signs should be attempted.

The chronic case

It is in the companion animals that most treatment of chronic disease is required. This does not mean that the process of chronic disease is different in farm animals – rather, that the purposes for which they are kept limit the opportunities for treating the conditions that arise. In the chronic case we are concerned with the survival of the individual animal, which in many ways is the antithesis of the farming situation. The first requirement is time. In chronic cases it is essential to consider all aspects at all levels, as the best prescriptions are those that are based on the totality of the symptoms. At least an hour should be allowed for the initial homeopathic consultation, sometimes longer. Follow-up consultations can also require more time than in the conventional situation, as it may be necessary to re-check ground already covered in order to be certain that the information on which the first prescription was made was correct. This is particularly important when there has not been the expected improvement in the case. It is, however, time well spent, as initially getting off in the right direction saves time later.

The exact technique of taking a case will vary with the individual veterinary surgeon, within certain basic guidelines. Some practitioners advocate the use of a questionnaire, to be filled in prior to the consultation. This has some attractions but can lead to a loss of flexibility in the approach; and unless time is spent working through the answers, to obtain the nuances that are so important in homeopathic prescribing, much information may be missed. A less rigid format from the start avoids this repetition, although some outline structure to the consultation is desirable to ensure that nothing is omitted.

The client should be allowed to play a major role in the consultation. A certain amount of direction is necessary but the veterinary surgeon should not orchestrate events. Avoid wherever possible putting words into the client's mouth, as there is an inbuilt tendency for them to agree with the person asking the question!

Most clients also have a tendency to avoid what they think will be a censure from the practitioner. Thus a question such as 'what is his/her favourite titbit?' may be met with the reply 'we never give any'. The truth may be very different, but there is the perception that veterinary surgeons do not approve of giving titbits (or pets sleeping on beds etc.) Make it clear that all revelations will be treated in a non-judgmental way.

Start with the family history. This is often a luxury in veterinary work as many animals are obtained without any meaningful family background. However, it is an aspect that should not be ignored, and it can be a useful factor in farm work where breeding patterns are tightly controlled. This can also be the case with companion animal breeders. Next should come the full medical and social history of the patient. Vaccinations, neutering, worming, flea treatments etc. are all important, as are details of reactions to any of those events. These can indicate possible aetiologies for the presenting condition or adverse effects on the immune system. If the start of the disease process can be traced to a particular event or set of circumstances, this should be investigated. It is an integral part of the whole picture and also opens up avenues of treatment. Previous accidents and/or illnesses must be noted. Do not confine the discussion to major incidents only – a fact such as minor wounds always healing slowly can be useful. Full details of all past and current conventional medication must also be obtained.

As mentioned above, it is important to include the mental aspects of the veterinary patients in the same way as the doctors do with human patients. While there are inevitably certain mental aspects that cannot be reliably ascertained, there is much that can be discovered. Hence enquiries about the personality of the patient must be part of veterinary case taking. This can be a difficult art, as it is necessary to allow the client to talk about their animal without indulging in sentimentality or wishful thinking. Questions such as 'How would you describe his/her temperament?' will often yield answers such as 'Lovely!' or 'Absolutely perfect!' which are not in themselves very helpful. However, it can on occasion be a useful starting point if followed up by questions concerning what the owner considers as lovely or perfect. Another approach is to present the client with hypothetical situations in which their animal might be found and ask them to describe how it would react. This allows the practitioner, with their knowledge of animal behaviour, to judge the temperament, and removes the tendency towards anthropomorphism. Thus instead of asking 'Is your dog aggressive towards other animals?' ask 'If your dog is approached by another dog while out walking, how will he react?'

Next come the 'generals'. These may be the most useful of the higher symptoms, as they can be easier to obtain in particular cases than the mentals. The general symptoms pertain to the patient in health just as much as in disease, although the effects, if any, of the illness on the general symptoms should be noted and considered.

Finally there are the local signs and symptoms. Many of these will be the signs that have been used to arrive at the conventional diagnosis. As common symptoms, in homeopathic terms they are of limited value. However, if a modality can be added to them, then they become useful local symptoms. Stiffness and pain in joints is a very common symptom in cases of arthritis but if it can be established that these are worse in damp weather, then the symptom becomes useful homeopathically.

The Herd/Flock/Kennel/Cattery Situation

Here the problem to be dealt with is either an acute disease affecting significant numbers of the group at one time, or an ongoing situation of acute cases occurring in individual animals. This latter is not a true chronic disease situation in either the homeopathic or the conventional sense, although it is often described as such.

In the first instance the affected group will be showing a range of symptoms, some of which will be common to all animals, some that will be exhibited by significant numbers but not by all of them, and some that will be confined to a small number or even individual members of the group. Individual case taking and treatment is usually impractical in these situations, and so the aim becomes to find a remedy that covers the broad range of symptoms being exhibited by the whole group. The common symptoms, as discussed above, are usually of limited value, and the main area to concentrate on will be the various symptoms being shown by sub-groups of animals within the whole. Combining these as if they came from only one animal will produce a remedy that, whilst not being the perfect individual match for every case, will be sufficiently close to be of benefit to the whole group. The more symptoms that can be included, of course, the closer will be the match. Hence it is still necessary to explore all the levels of symptoms as described above, although in practice the locals will probably be more represented than the mentals and generals.

In the second situation, while individual animals can be dealt with as acute cases and given specific prescriptions, there will be some underlying factor which must be investigated and addressed. This may of course be a pure management fault, which needs correction as in any conventional treatment approach. There is however the possibility of more homeopathically-orientated factors being involved, for example miasmatic influences, and these must be addressed if the situation is to be successfully resolved.

The case taking in these situations will of necessity veer towards the local signs, although compared to the true acute condition the family, social, and medical history of the group assumes a greater significance, and causality often assumes a major role. For example, movement of stock in the course of routine management may be unavoidable, but it may also be a trigger in the appearance of the disease pattern. As such movements cannot be avoided, because of the intrinsic nature of the commercial system, they must be taken into account in the selection of the remedy.

The mental and general symptoms of individual animals should not be ignored, but utilised as and if appropriate. If the majority of a group show similar mental characteristics, for example highly strung or docile, then this feature becomes relevant in the search for the correct remedy.

It is possible in appropriate circumstances to deal with a whole herd as if it was one single animal. Here the case is taken by selecting signs that are representative of both the disease pattern and background nature of the group, although they may not be present in every animal. The remedy thus selected will go a long way towards covering the whole disease picture. This is similar to the approach outlined for the true acute situation, but takes a greater account of factors influencing the problem on a broader and deeper front.

Pitfalls and Interpretation

In acquiring information it must always be remembered that the prescriber is working through a third party, either the owner or handler/keeper. In some instances this may enhance the information, as with a stockman who really knows his animals. In others there may be a very subjective owner's interpretation of what is observed, and this can be misleading. Anthropomorphism is a constant hazard in the mental sphere, as is a transference of the owner's emotions onto the interpretation that is placed on the animal's behaviour. The fact that the environment in which the animal lives is based on the requirements and desires of the owner adds a further complication. It may be reported that an animal does not sit near to a fire or radiator if the opportunity occurs, but this cannot automatically be interpreted as a dislike of heat. The house may be kept warm to meet the owner's requirements, and the animal may in fact have a degree of liking for heat which is being met by the background temperature. A symptom of dislike of heat can only be considered if the animal makes positive moves to seek cooler places. Similarly, an animal that prefers to be cool may be prepared to remain near a source of heat if the owner, from whom it craves attention, remains seated near the heat. Wherever possible, judgements about mental and general symptoms should not be made on one feature alone. The owner's susceptibility to advertising and/or their religious or philosophical beliefs may well govern the diet of the animal. The major effect here is usually to limit the dietary information that we have available; in some cases a poor diet will constitute an obstacle to the body's response to the remedy.

In ascertaining the modalities at a more local level, the situation is often not as clear-cut as it may at first appear. It could emerge that an irritation is < (worse) in the evening. This can in fact be the time modality that it appears to be. However, the irritation may also vary for the following reasons:

- It is only in the evening that the owner is settled enough to observe the animal. It may also be that the scratching annoys them more at that time because they are trying to relax. In this instance there is in fact no modality.

- As the owner is sitting relaxing, they may have increased the level of heating in the house. Hence what we are dealing with here is a heat modality.

- The animal may have been fed in the evening and this has increased the irritation.

- The animal may be played with and touched more at this time, and this is increasing the irritation.

In spite of the above it is possible to obtain a lot of relevant and useful information in most cases. The next problem is how to interpret it in order to maximise its benefit.

Signs and symptoms are weighted in order of importance as indicated above, from the rare and peculiar, through the mentals and generals, to the locals. In an ideal case there will be symptoms from all levels involved in the analysis, but of necessity there will be occasions when this is not possible, and use must be made of what is available. It may be necessary to start treatment without a complete remedy picture, and this must be accepted on occasion. A remedy correctly chosen on the picture presented, albeit incomplete, will often be the 'similar' rather than the simillimum, and this will be enough to produce changes in the picture, which will enable a more accurate choice to be made for the second prescription.

A major difficulty in interpretation is the effect of conventional medication on the presenting picture. The use of NSAIDs in cases of arthritis will often prevent the manifestation of the true pattern of the locomotor difficulties that would otherwise be present in the picture. The modality of being either better (>) or worse (<) for movement is particularly useful in such cases, but in those that are receiving medication this valuable information may be unobtainable. In extreme cases the true picture may be completely suppressed by the current medication, and no accurate prescribing can be undertaken until the underlying situation can be revealed. In cases where the withdrawal of conventional medication would lead to the re-appearance of unacceptable symptoms, as in epilepsy where the convulsions are completely controlled, then initial assessment of the case must rest on mental, general, or concomitant symptoms that form no part of the conventional picture. In other cases the presenting picture will be a combination of genuine and drug-induced symptoms (their side effects) and these must be separated.

Occasionally, however, the effects of medication can help in interpretation. If the case history reveals that the patient does not drink much and that the administration of corticosteroids does not increase the thirst, then this would lend weight to the inclusion of 'thirstless' as a general symptom in the case.

True 'strange, rare, and peculiar'symptoms are, by definition, not all that common and are like gold dust when they can be found and used. Symptoms such as the case of a cat that developed a leather fetish at the time of the onset of the apparently unrelated illness, and who would lie on it, play with it or lick and eat it at every opportunity!

At the same time, unexpected or unusual reactions can lead to a particular symptom being given greater consideration than would otherwise be the case. With a full-coated breed of dog, for example, more emphasis will be placed on a strong liking for heat than would be the case with a short-haired breed such as a whippet. Similarly, fear of noise in a gun dog will be of significance.

Also, points about a case which the owner brings out very strongly *without prompting* are potentially of greater significance than those which have to be almost forced out of them.

One danger to be avoided is the assumption that all animals of a particular breed are alike in their mental and general symptoms. This is particularly important when the constitutional remedy (Chapter 9) is being considered. While it is true that members of the same breed do share a number of features which may correspond to a particular remedy, there will always be exceptions and variations in intensity. The soft, affectionate nature of most golden retrievers, or the exuberance of the Irish setter, may match the remedies Pulsatilla and Phosphorus respectively, but all members of those breeds cannot be assumed to be of the appropriate type. Breed characteristics must always be taken into account, but the more typical the feature, the less emphasis should be given to it. The more a feature diverges from the typical, the more significant it becomes. A pit bull terrier that was afraid of all other dogs would be very significant.

Miasmatic and Constitutional Symptoms

These are not further types of symptoms, but represent a different method of classification of those described above. After a case has been taken there will be some of the symptoms which, when taken together, reveal a definite pattern that points towards either a particular constitutional type or a miasmatic influence. Both may be present in the same case, as the two concepts overlap to some degree. The concept of the constitution and how this is employed in practice is dealt with in Chapter 9. For the moment it is sufficient to describe it as a broad-based interpretation of the patient's underlying type. Symptoms from the mental and general levels are most commonly involved in this, and considerations of bodily conformation are also relevant. A strong liking for heat will point towards certain remedies, while a strong aversion to it will suggest others. Similarly, a heavily built conformation will bring emphasis to remedies that would not rate so highly in a fine-boned animal.

It must be stressed however that the choice of remedy should never be made on the basis of one sign or symptom alone, but always by using the full range of information that is available.

Miasmatic symptoms are indications of particular types of reaction on the part of the body that point to one of the miasmatic influences. Signs and symptoms that indicate one of these processes at work are termed miasmatic symptoms. Within the hierarchy of symptoms they can be found at any level, but what is of value in prescribing is when the symptoms point to a degree of dominance in the activity of one particular miasm.

The concepts of constitutional and miasmatic symptoms may be considered to lie more in the field of interpretation than that of basic information gathering, but it is important to bear them in mind during the case-taking process.

Observation

All the above is in addition to normal conventional case taking, and a full physical examination of the patient is essential. In addition to its conventional scope, the examination can yield information of purely homeopathic relevance. Irrespective of the presenting condition, the fact that, for example, the patient exhibits a general redness around the body orifices will be an indication for the use of a particular remedy (Sulphur).

Observation is a key element in the case-taking procedure, and it is a mistake to wait until the patient is in the consulting room before beginning the process. In appropriate species the first observation should be of the animal in the waiting room, or even on its way into the building. With species that are confined, such as cats, information can be obtained from the behaviour of the animal in its basket and its reaction to being removed from it. The behaviour in these situations can give useful clues. Once in the consulting room, the ideal is for the animal to be allowed freedom to roam while the case is being talked about. In this way the veterinary surgeon can make his or her own judgement regarding the temperament, which together with the owner's assessment builds up to a reliable picture. Observation of the animal in its own environment can be useful on occasion. Although modern practice organisation tends to be against this, the 'home visit' can yield valuable information and should not be dismissed by the homeopathic veterinary surgeon.

On the physical plane too, direct observation is a great aid, and can help to overcome the subjective interpretations of the owner. In homeopathic prescribing the exact nature of discharges and the exact appearance of pathology is important. The veterinary surgeon's own assessment of the colour of a discharge, or the hardness of a lump, greatly increases both the potential accuracy of the prescription and the assessment of progress. An individual soon learns to equate their evaluation of a particular symptom against the descriptions given in the standard reference works, and as a result is able to introduce a degree of consistency into what may otherwise become a confusing situation.

Conventional Investigations and Diagnosis

It is in interpreting the information obtained from case taking and investigation that some of the differences between the systems occur.

The conventional world uses the information to standardise and classify the situation into a diagnosis, which revolves around giving a name to a particular disease process. At the other end of the scale is the approach of some homeopaths, summed up in the phrase 'The name of your disease is of no interest to me, and the name of your remedy is of no interest to you'.

Conventionally, the diagnosis determines entirely the nature and direction of the treatment. Homeopathically, it is only a starting point from which the prescriber refers back to the patient to arrive at the treatment. But it is a starting point and must not be ignored.

At the heart of this difference is the basic divergence in the concept of disease which has already been discussed. The conventional approach regards the signs and to a lesser degree the symptoms as the disease itself. Homeopathically the signs are regarded as the end products of the disease process, with the symptoms being largely indicative of that process in the individual. Conventionally, pathology causes malfunction; homeopathically, malfunction causes pathology. Pathological findings are only another part of the total symptom picture, the whole of which is a manifestation of the functional imbalance in the patient's system.

This difference also applies in the more acute situations. Where a conventional practitioner will think in terms of a case of distemper, essentially like every other case and to be dealt with accordingly, the homeopath will think of it as a form of distemper which is unique to that patient, with variations of colour and quantities of discharges, exact nature of the diarrhoea, worsening at particular times of day, and other individualising features; and the choice of remedy for that patient will be arrived at by reference to those individual manifestation of the disease. (Details of how this information is analysed are discussed in the next chapter.)

The difference is purely one of perspective, with no dispute about the usefulness of all the available information. The incorporation of the conventional diagnosis as part of the whole picture is an integral part of modern homeopathic practice, and is the baseline from which the individualisation is built. The conventional diagnosis reveals much about the disease process which has to be known, but if it is adhered to rigidly it rapidly becomes a straightjacket.

Hahnemann advanced his ideas and clarified the homeopathic approach in an age before most of the diagnostic aids that are nowadays taken for granted had been developed. The concepts concerning bacteria and infection had not been advanced, although Hahnemann himself predicted them ('Cure and Prevention of Asiatic Cholera', 1831; in *Lesser Writings*, 1851) some 80 years before Pasteur and Koch developed the ideas that became Germ Theory. Although there is no mention of such matters in the original writings and provings, it does not mean that there is any intrinsic antagonism or incompatibility between the modern developments and homeopathy. Homeopathy's core concept of 'like cures like' implies that it is desirable to know everything possible about both the disease and the remedy. The essential difference between the two systems is that the conventional world bases its therapeutics on not requiring the practitioner to know everything about the individual aspects of a case.

In Paragraph 14 of the *Organon* Hahnemann wrote: 'There is nothing curably diseased, nor any curable, invisible disease alteration in the human interior that, by disease signs and symptoms would not present itself to the exactly observing physician for discernment.' In the next paragraph he writes: 'The suffering of the morbidly mistuned, spirit-like *dynamis* (life force) enlivening our body in the invisible interior, and the complex of the outwardly perceptible symptoms portraying the present malady, which are organised by the dynamis in the organism, form a whole.'

Although referring to humans, Hahnemann's ideas apply just as much to animals, and when it is realised that it is now possible to 'see' into the interior of the body, to a degree unimagined in Hahnemann's day, it is clear that there is no intrinsic difficulty in reconciling modern developments with basic homeopathic philosophy. The results of all the modern diagnostic techniques are in accord with Hahnemann's concept of the totality of symptoms. The knowledge derived from investigative procedures is being added to the remedy pictures and as a result is broadening their usefulness.

References

Clover, A. (1989) *Homeopathy Reconsidered*. London: Victor Gollancz.

Kaplan, B. (2001) *The Homeopathic Conversation*. London: Natural Medicine Press.

Saxton, J.G.G. (1998) Diagnosis, the love-hate relationship. *Proceedings of the LIGA Conference*, Amsterdam.

Chapter 7

Matching the Symptoms

The Materia Medica

Having obtained the symptoms of the case, as discussed in Chapter 6, it is necessary to find a homeopathic remedy whose symptomatology matches them as closely as possible.

This information is contained in the multitude of reference works which constitute the homeopathic materia medica. This large body of work is constantly being revised, updated and added to as existing remedies are more closely studied and new remedies investigated.

Hahnemann's *Fragmenta De Viribus Medicamentorum Positivis* and *Materia Medica Pura* consisted entirely of lists of symptoms obtained in provings, all carried out using material doses of the remedies. However, his *Chronic Diseases* lists symptoms of provings carried out using the 30th centesimal potency.

The first English contribution to the homeopathic materia medica came with Hughes' *Cyclopaedia of Drug Pathogenesy*, published in 1884. Hughes was deeply sceptical of both Hahnemann and the higher potencies, and took it on himself to expunge from the materia medica all but the toxic and material drug symptoms from healthy provers. Other authors began to emphasise those symptoms that had been found to be useful in clinical practice, and perhaps the most influential of these was Hering, whose *Guiding Symptoms of our Materia Medica* was published in 1879; this set out the information in a way that was easier to read, and indicated the most well-verified symptoms. This attempt at making the materia medica more easily usable and more accessible was followed by others, such as H.C. Allen. His *Keynotes* lists in no more than a couple of small pages the principal features of a remedy, with bold type emphasising the most characteristic symptoms.

The great English homeopath Clarke published his 3-volume *Dictionary of Materia Medica* in 1900. This is a compilation of information from other authors, as well as Clarke's own experience, and his inclusion of anecdotes from practice helps to make it far more readable than some of the earlier works.

However, it was Kent more than anyone else who made the hugely important step of describing a remedy in a narrative style which allowed the reader to build up a picture of the patient requiring that remedy. His *Lectures on Materia Medica* (1904) is still a standard work. Kent's style was expanded by Tyler in her *Homoeopathic Drug Pictures,* which is written in such a way that it has been the bed-time reading of many aspiring homeopaths. Gibson's *Studies of Homoeopathic Remedies* is similarly readable. This type of work increasingly emphasises the mental symptoms of the remedies, and the psychoanalytical approach is taken further by Vithoulkas in his *Essences*, by Coulter in her *Portraits of Homeopathic Medicines*, and by Bailey in his *Homeopathic Psychology.* These latter in particular provide ways of understanding the remedies in a psychological way which, once grasped, can act as a framework for remembering more of the details of the drug picture.

Sankaran uses a similar approach in his *Soul of Homeopathy,* but one where the remedy states are each perceived as corresponding to a basic delusion which directs the patient into his or her behaviour. While it is perhaps difficult to apply this to animals, nevertheless the under-standing of the remedies gained can be of great help in veterinary prescribing. Yet another approach has been developed by Jan Scholten, who has studied the periodic table of the elements and allotted characteristics to each element depending on its position therein. In the light of this he postulates – with remarkable accuracy – the therapeutic properties of salts and minerals by studying their component cations and anions. His books *Homeopathy and Minerals* and *Homeopathy and the Elements* discuss these concepts in depth.

Several attempts have been made at reducing the information in the materia medica to a size which allows ready reference, in the style of *Keynotes.* Boericke's *Pocket Manual of Homœopathic Materia Medica* (1927) has a useful preamble to each remedy which sets the scene for the information that follows. The rest of the information is set out succinctly, with italic script to emphasise those symptoms which are most characteristic of the remedy. Phatak's *Materia Medica of Homoeopathic Medicines* (1977) is similar, but as befits a more modern work is more expansive on the mental symptoms.

Morrison's *Desktop Guide to Keynotes and Confirmatory Signs* (1993) is a more recent and therefore up-to-date example.

In recent years Franz Vermeulen has combined most of the significant texts to create a *Concordant Materia Medica*, and this may justifiably be considered the standard text of homeopathic materia medica at present. In addition, his more recent work *Prisma* emphasises the parallels between homeopathic drug pictures and the substances from which they are derived. This indeed aids the modern-thinking homeopath to understand the remedies more fully.

It can be seen that the homeopathic materia medica has evolved from Hahnemann's time to the present day from a simple, unstructured list of symptoms experienced by provers of material doses of substances, into approaches which allow the student to grasp a single salient concept for a particular remedy, around which an understanding of it can be built. This makes the study of homeopathic materia medica not only more interesting, but ultimately a lot easier. Different approaches appeal to different individuals and the more recent and very diverse insights into the materia medica such as those by Vithoulkas, Scholten and Sankaran allow a great deal of flexibility in how one studies, understands and ultimately uses the remedies. However, even today's imaginative descriptions of the homeopathic materia medica are based squarely on the classical triad of provings, toxicological studies and clinical experience. It is only in this way that the materia medica can stand the test of time as a reliable source of information for the practising homeopath.

Veterinary Materia Medica

Very little information exists on veterinary homeopathic materia medica. Until recently the only such work to date was a slim volume entitled *A Veterinary Materia Medica* by George Macleod. Unfortunately, it is of such brevity and the information of such a pathological nature that it is of limited use to the serious student of veterinary homeopathy. Useful materia medica sections are contained in Day's *Homoeopathic Treatment of Small Animals* and other similar books, but the descriptions are generally necessarily brief. Don Hamilton's *Homeopathic Care for Cats and Dogs* contains a useful materia medica section and Atjo Westerhuis' *Your Dog and Homeopathy* has an excellent chapter on 'homeopathic types'. However, the International Association for Veterinary Homeopathy has for some years been developing a *Homeopathic Materia Medica Veterinaria* and the first volume, as yet only in French and German, is now available. This project is perhaps the most promising for veterinary surgeons, but no doubt as veterinary homeopathy continues to develop along similar lines to its medical counterpart, more purely veterinary information will be published.

In the meantime, the human homeopathic materia medica provides ample information for veterinary prescribing. With a little experience it is quite easy to interpret human symptomatology in veterinary terms, and with a little imagination even some of the more complex concepts such as emotional states and delusions can be useful to the veterinary homeopath.

The Repertories

The development of the materia medica to the present position helps us to understand the remedies more easily and more fully, but still leaves us with a great deal of work to do before we can even attempt to match our patient's symptoms with those of a homeopathic remedy.

Hahnemann himself recognised the need for some way of matching a given symptom with a remedy and the second part of his *Fragmenta* consisted of an index of symptoms, or 'repertory', whereby any particular symptom could be matched to those remedies which were appropriate. A repertory is therefore a reference key which lists symptoms under headings (termed 'rubrics'). Under each rubric is a list of all the remedies which are appropriate to that symptom. For instance the rubric 'Mind; anxiety; in a crowd' contains 11 remedies in the fifth edition of *Synthesis*. The rubric 'Stomach; pain; drinking, after' contains 31 remedies. If several rubrics are taken, representing the important symptoms of a case, analysis of them will show that some remedies appear in most, if not all, of the rubrics, while others only appear in one or two rubrics. The remedies which appear in most of the rubrics will be those most likely to be indicated in that case. The final choice within the shortlist will depend on reference to the materia medica.

The repertory therefore provides a simple way of narrowing down the choice of remedy and pointing the way towards the remedy best indicated for the case. Many such works followed Hahnemann's, notably von Boenninghausen's *Repertory of the Antipsoric Remedies* (1833) and Constantine Lippe's *Repertory to the More Characteristic Symptoms of the Materia Medica* (1880). However, once again it was Kent who developed the repertory into an essential and practical part of homeopathic prescribing. Like von Boenninghausen before him, he graded the remedies within a rubric, depending on how significant he considered them to be for the symptom represented. In his *Repertory of the Homoeopathic Materia Medica* (1899) bold type denotes the greatest significance, italics intermediate and plain type the least significance. Kent's *Repertory* has since been extensively corrected and expanded, as for instance in Künzli's *Kent's Repertorium Generale* (1987), but it remains the basis for most modern repertories. A legacy of this is that much of the terminology of the repertory remains somewhat archaic and a necessary part of learning to use it involves getting used to the rather old-fashioned language. In practice however this is not generally a handicap.

The organisation within Kent's repertory follows broadly anatomical lines. The first chapter is headed 'Mind', the next 'Head' and subsequent chapters deal with other anatomical parts or systems in a fairly logical sequence. The last chapter deals with 'Generals' and includes most of the modalities. The layout within a particular chapter follows a precise order, largely alphabetical, though in certain areas a different order is used. For instance, sub-rubrics of a symptom generally follow the order of: time, other modalities, location, character. Thus in the chapter 'Rectum', under the rubric 'Diarrhoea', 'Evening' comes before 'Coffee, after', and in the chapter 'Head', the rubric 'Pain; sleep; ameliorates' comes before 'Pain; forehead, in', which comes before 'Pain; stitching'. This format has found almost universal use, and is that used in *Synthesis*, although Murphy (1993) uses an alphabetical order for the body systems, considering this to be more logical and easier to use. Murphy has also added many new chapters and uses terminology which is more modern. Examples of new chapter headings include 'Children', 'Environment', 'Shoulders' and 'Ankles' (the latter both being included in 'Extremities' in the Kentian system).

Kent's grading approach lends the repertory to a numerical 'scoring' system. If bold type remedies are given the score 3, italics 2 and plain type 1, the addition of these scores from several rubrics provides a figure which represents the potential importance of that remedy to the case. Each remedy thus has a score on two counts; the number of rubrics in which it is represented, and the sum of the numerical scores from each rubric. A remedy should be considered if it has a high score on both of these counts. However, it should be stressed that repertorisation and case analysis in this way will only provide a list of likely remedies, and no prescription should be made on repertorisation alone. If rubrics have been well chosen, the indicated remedy should be present among the top half dozen or so remedies, but it needs to be repeated that the final choice should only be made after reference to the materia medica.

The mechanics of doing this manually can be devised using a piece of graph paper: the rubrics are written at the top of the columns and the names of the remedies down the left hand side. The scores are entered in the appropriate squares and totals are produced by adding up the figures for each remedy on the lateral scale. Printed sheets are available with all the common remedies already filled in and spaces left for any others which come up in the repertorisation.

The table overleaf shows a simplified example of the repertorisation of the case of a terrier-cross dog suffering from atopic dermatitis. The patient was extremely fastidious in maintaining the pristine cleanliness of his appearance; he was restless at night, was extremely chilly and had an increased thirst, but for small quantities at a time. A concomitant symptom was a nervous twitch of the limbs which came on as he was falling asleep. The pruritus was so severe that the dog would frequently make himself bleed, and there was marked flaking of the lesions. All the symptoms were worse when the patient was taken to the seaside.

The repertorisation reveals a clear first choice of Arsenicum Album, and this effected a complete cure of all symptoms. However, this case has been chosen simply as an example of the mechanics of repertorisation; in practice, the choice of remedy is likely to be found by comparing the materia medica of the leading four or five remedies, and it is rare for the result to be as clear-cut as in this example. The repertorisation chart has similarly been simplified and would normally include more remedies, though even then only the most common homeopathic remedies would be printed; the spaces in the table allow the addition of further remedies as may be necessary for any particular case.

Such full analysis of the case may not always be necessary; depending on the skill and experience of the prescriber it may only be necessary to look up two or three well-selected rubrics which together represent the essence of the case, or indeed the one rubric which is essential to the case. Conversely, the prescriber may simply need to refer to the rubric with which they are not familiar, to find the required remedy. These shorter approaches necessitate a high degree of experience and knowledge of the materia medica to yield consistent results – however, used in this way the repertory can be a tool for ready and quick reference in the consulting room, just as much as a means of deep analysis of a case.

Computer Repertories

To perform a full analysis manually is extremely time-consuming, and from as early as 1892 several attempts were made to facilitate it using systems of punched cards. The advent of computer technology has resulted in an enormous leap in repertorisation techniques. Cara, Radar and MacRepertory (originally developed for Apple Macintosh, but also available for PCs) are market leaders and are all widely used. Radar is available in book form, under the title of *Synthesis*. Each system has its own unique characteristics and each distributor will offer a variety of packages to suit the individual prescriber.

Computer programmes allow innovative and imaginative analysis regimes and allow such techniques as the weighting of symptoms to be used. For instance, a symptom which is clearly marked in the patient, and which seems to be of major importance – perhaps a 'strange, rare and peculiar' (SRP) – may be weighted 4 whereas a symptom which is common or not clearly marked in the patient may be weighted 1. The weighting of 4 would bias the analysis towards that symptom. This permits the patient's individual disease state to be more accurately represented by the repertorisation.

There are other ways in which computer repertories can yield more accurate results than their manual equivalents. For instance it is common for the 'polychrests' ('large' remedies which cover a wide spectrum of symptoms) to dominate the results of the analysis; any 'smaller' remedies which may be useful to the case may be missed. Computer repertorisation allows the polychrests to be suppressed, thus allowing the smaller remedies to come to the attention of the homeopath. Various advisory systems may also be included in a package, such as Radar's 'Vithoulkas Expert System', which uses the experience of George Vithoulkas to direct investigations if the result of the repertorisation does not present a sufficiently clear choice of remedy.

As with any computer system, the benefits are proportional to the quality of the information fed into the system, and indeed this applies to repertorisation generally. It is far better to use a few well-chosen rubrics, whose significance to the case is unquestioned, rather than a lot of rubrics which are of a general or highly subjective nature. Such rubrics as 'Stomach; thirst' (with 378 remedies in Radar) or 'Stomach; appetite; wanting' (307 remedies) are of virtually no value whatsoever in individualising a case, whereas such rubrics as 'Generals;

Sample Repertorisation

1 Mind – Fastidious
2 Mind – Restlessness after midnight
3 Generals – Lack of vital heat
4 Generals – Air seaside; air at the, aggravates
5 Stomach – Thirst small quantities and often
6 Extremities – Twitching on falling asleep
7 Skin – Itching; must scratch until it bleeds
8 Skin – Eruptions desquamating

Remedy	1	2	3	4	5	6	7	8	Totals
Aconitum		1	1			1		1	3/3
Aloe									
Alumina	1		3			2	1		7/4
Antim. Crud.			2						
Antim. Tart.								1	
Apis			2	2				1	6/3
Argent. Nit.	1		2						
Arnica									
Arsen. Alb.	3	3	2	2		3	3	2	**18/8**
Aurum	1		2					2	
Baryta Carb.			3				2	1	6/3
Belladonna						2		3	
Bryonia		1		1					

Remedy	1	2	3	4	5	6	7	8	Totals
Ignatia									3/3
Ipecac.			2						
Iodum	1			1				1	3/3
Kali Bich.	1		3						
Kali Carb.	2		3		1				6/3
Lachesis			2					1	
Lycopodium	1	1	2		1				5/4
Mag. Carb.			1			1		2	4/3
Merc. Corr.							2	1	
Merc. Sol.	1		2					2	5/3

Sample Repertorisation (continued)

Remedy	1	2	3	4	6	7	8	Totals
Calc. Carb.			3		1		2	6/3
Calc. Fluor.			2					
Calc. Phos.	1		3					6/3
Cantharis							1	
Causticum	2		3				1	
Chamomilla	1				2		1	
Colchicum			2					
Colocynth						2	2	
Cuprum	1			1			1	
Drosera								
Dulcamara			3				2	
Ferrum			3				1	
Gelsemium								
Graphites	2		3		2		2	9/4

Remedy	1	2	3	4	5	6	7	8	Totals
Nat. Mur.	2		2	3		2		1	**10/5**
Nat. Sulph.	1								
Nit. Ac.		2	3				1		6/3
Nux Vom.	2		3						
Phosphorus	1		3				1	2	7/4
Psorinum			3				2	3	8/3
Pulsatilla	1				1	1	2	2	7/5
Rhus Tox.		3	3	2	1			2	**11/5**
Sepia	1		2	3				3	9/4
Silica	1	1	3	1				2	8/5
Staphysagria	1		2					2	5/3
Sulphur	1	1	2		2			2	8/5
Thuja	1		3					1	5/3
Tub. Bov.			2	2	1				5/3

emaciation; appetite with emaciation; ravenous' (35 remedies) or 'Extremities; pain; motion amel.' (35 remedies) would be of far greater value. 'Stomach; thirstless – accompanied by: Mouth; dryness of' (a 'strange, rare and peculiar' and with two remedies only) would rate as even more useful. Three or four rubrics such as these latter three could well be sufficient for an accurate repertorisation. Of course, the temptation to use several rubrics is far greater with computer repertorisation than when the process has to be laboriously carried out with pencil and paper! For this reason it is recommended that the student of homeopathy initially practices repertorisation manually. This will encourage the development of the skill to select rubrics which truly represent the individuality of the case.

Wherever possible a homeopathic prescription is based on the totality of symptoms presented, and for this reason it is generally accepted that an accurate repertorisation should include a range of mental, general and local symptoms. Consideration of how clearly each symptom is represented in the patient, and how important each one is in accurately reflecting the individual disease state in that particular patient, will allow the symptoms to be carefully weighted. This will further refine the process of repertorisation with a consequent improvement in the accuracy of the analysis.

An extension of computer analysis is the creation of programmes such as MacRepertory's *Reference Works* or Radar's *Encyclopedia Homeopathica*, which scan the materia medica itself. The repertories by their very nature must lag behind the materia medica in incorporating new information; it is only recently, for instance that all the information contained in Boericke's *Pocket Manual* has been incorporated into a repertory programme, and some workers feel that the repertory may eventually be succeeded by the materia medica search programmes.

Veterinary Repertories

In the same way that veterinarians have adapted their use of the human materia medica to suit their needs, so it is with the repertory. There are parts which the veterinary homeopath cannot make use of, for instance all the sections on character of pain, and there is a difficulty when considering the relevance of rubrics appertaining to such anatomical differences as 'hands' and 'feet' compared to 'front feet' and 'hooves'. However, it is possible to make use of the human repertory, and Kent's repertory and its successors have for many years been invaluable to the veterinary homeopath. There is nevertheless no doubt that a repertory created specifically for veterinary homeopaths is required.

Macleod's *Veterinary Materia Medica* contains a small repertory, and most of the popular books on the homeopathic treatment of animals are laid out in a style similar to the repertory, but as yet there is no major work in this field. Matthew Glencross combines information from several veterinary texts in his *Veterinary Repertory*, published as part of *Therapeutics of Veterinary Homeopathy* by B.P. Madrewar, but this is still very rudimentary. An exciting development therefore, in 2001, was the release of Radar's veterinary programme. This consists of the medical programme with veterinary additions, and many prominent veterinary homeopaths from around the world are now contributing to this enormously important project. It may not be long before there exists a repertory which is tailored specifically to the needs of the veterinary homeopath.

Other Levels of Prescribing

While repertorisation on the totality of the case represents homeopathic prescribing in its most sophisticated form, it is by no means the only way of finding a suitable remedy for a particular patient. Other methods of achieving an effective prescription are:

Local prescribing

Here a prescription is made on local signs alone. Preferably there should be at least one clear modality, but even where this is not possible, homeopathy can be usefully employed at this level.

Example: A Jack Russell terrier suffering from arthritis which is worse in cold and damp weather and better for continued movement receives Rhus Toxicodendron, based on the local symptoms and modalities.

Organ-specific prescribing

Many homeopathic medicines have known effects which are limited to, or particularly marked in, a particular organ. Where the specific pathology in a patient corresponds, this form of prescribing can be applied most usefully. Renal and hepatic diseases are areas where this approach is commonly used.

Example: A New Forest pony suffering from chronic liver disease receives Chelidonium Majus, as this remedy is known to have a beneficial effect on the liver.

Pathological prescribing

Here, it is the pathological process which is the guiding principle. Thus there are remedies which are particularly appropriate for haemorrhage, fever or bruising where the pathology exactly mirrors the remedy picture.

Example: A domestic shorthair cat involved in a road accident and suffering from multiple contusions receives Arnica Montana, a specific remedy for bruising.

Functional prescribing

This is a form of local prescribing which considers the regulation of function of an organ. For example, where the predominating functional upset is spasm, a particular group of medicines that have spasm as a marked feature may be considered. Similarly, a particular organ may be malfunctioning, and a homeopathic medicine may be employed in a regulatory manner to rectify this.

Example: A greyhound suffering from attacks of cramp receives Cuprum Metallicum, a remedy in which spasm is a major feature.

Proven indications

The wealth of experience which has, and continues to be, built up within both human and veterinary homeopathy can be usefully employed by noting which remedies have been used successfully in any particular condition. Certain workers may have found that a particular condition has frequently responded to certain remedies, and this can be a useful way of shortlisting medicines. The majority of the remedies cited in the second section of this book have been selected on this basis. It should be remembered also that information on areas of disease beyond the presenting complaint (the 'concomitant symptoms') can also be used in this way.

Example: A Light Hunter horse suffering from ragwort poisoning receives Lycopodium Clavatum, a remedy which has been found useful in this condition.

Causality

One of the simplest and most direct ways of remedy selection involves taking note of the cause of the disease. The repertories contain such rubrics as 'Mind; ailments from; grief', and 'Generals; wet; getting', and where the cause of onset of the condition is known this can be a rapid way of finding the right remedy for a patient. An extension of this is the so-called 'Never Well Since' syndrome (NWS). These words are often used by clients reporting on their animals – if such a phenomenon can be identified, treatment of that condition as if it were still present can lead to a successful outcome.

Example: An adult Siamese cat who is depressed and inappetant following the loss of its littermate receives Ignatia Amara, one of the major remedies for grief.

Keynotes

A keynote symptom is one which is so clear and specific that it points to a very small number of remedies, or even a single one. A keynote symptom may be a local, general or mental symptom, or indeed a modality. It may also be something less concrete and represent a general theme of a remedy.

Example: A Border Collie bitch who has suffered a sudden paralysis receives Phosphorus, based on the keynote 'sudden onset'.

The predominant miasm

Identifying which **miasm** predominates in a patient can also help to reduce the number of possible remedies in a case. Using Hahnemann's original three miasms alone will reduce the remedy shortlist correspondingly; indeed, as we shall see in Chapters 11 and 12, a sufficiently strong miasmatic pattern in a patient may indicate the use of the appropriate miasmatic 'nosode' as an effective remedy.

Example: A dog suffering from atopy received Tuberculinum Bovinum as the symptom picture corresponds to the tubercular miasm.

Taxonomic class of remedy

It has long been noted that remedies may be classified depending on their source material; categorising the patient into a remedy type showing features of 'plant, animal or inorganic' material can be a useful starting point. Further classification on taxonomic grounds can also be of immense value, and much work continues to be done in this field. Scholten's work on the periodic table and Sankaran's on families such as the Ranunculaceae or the snake venom remedies are but two examples of this approach.

Example: An old terrier-cross dog who keeps his owners awake at night by barking receives Cenchris Contortrix, a snake venom remedy. The dog is animated and competitive, characteristics of animal remedies, and is jealous and suspicious, characteristics of snake remedies.

Constitutional prescribing

Here the prescription depends not only on the symptoms present, but also relies heavily on the basic physical and mental characteristics of the patient. Further discussion of this concept is contained in Chapter 9.

Example: A Jersey cow suffering from endometritis receives Pulsatilla Nigricans. The cow is mild, gentle, yielding, affectionate and thirstless – characteristics of the Pulsatilla constitutional type.

Finally it should be noted that while all of the above are valid ways of finding the correct remedy for a particular patient, they are only aids. The final decision should only be made after extensive reference to the materia medica.

Chapter 8

Practical Prescribing

Recognising the Problem

The first stage in prescribing is to decide on the exact nature of the condition to be treated, as this will have an influence on both the potency selected and the frequency of administration. The first type of case is the acute or per-acute, of sudden onset, and in many instances presenting a threat to the survival of the patient. Within this group there is of course a gradation with regard to the urgency of the situation, but in general terms prompt action is required. Infections, poisonings, injuries etc. fall into this group. At the other extreme is the chronic condition, of slower onset and, in homeopathic terms often presenting signs of the involvement of several different body systems. Between these two will be met the acute flare-up of an underlying chronic condition.

The acute case will require the use of either one or a small number of remedies over a short timescale. In an ideal world only one remedy will be needed, and in individual animals and groups of both companion and farm animals suffering from epizootic diseases this should be possible, due to the predominant effect of the pathogen producing a narrow range of symptoms. In some cases it may not always be possible to identify clearly the simillimum with the information available, and time is not on the prescriber's side. The use of two remedies at the same time is thus acceptable in practice, although they should not be given in the same mouthful. An interval should always be allowed, ideally at least ten minutes, although this may not be possible.

The use of remedies to aid recovery following injury and/or surgery, although part of an acute picture, often entails repeating remedies over a somewhat longer period of time. In cases of enzootic disease the individual constitution(s) of the animal(s) will influence the symptom picture to a greater extent than in the epizootic situation. In a group of animals it may thus not be possible to find one remedy that covers the whole picture. In these cases it may be necessary to utilise two or possibly three remedies in total to produce in effect a 'group simillimum', with all the selected remedies being given concurrently. These remedies will all have been selected based on aspects of the group symptom picture and will thus have pictures that are in some ways similar and overlapping, but the focus of their activity will be slightly different, with the overlap occurring away from the keynotes and major features of each. This may be represented as:

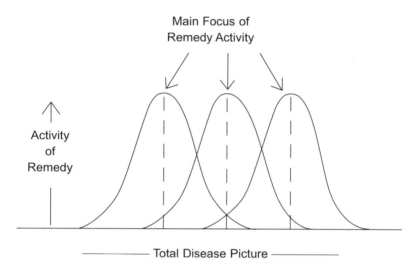

Main Focus of
Remedy Activity

Activity
of
Remedy

Total Disease Picture

In the chronic case a somewhat similar approach involves the use of possibly a number of remedies in succession over a more protracted timescale. The acute flare-up in the course of a chronic disease is dealt with essentially as an acute disease, with the difference that the life-threatening element is usually not present.

Dosage Considerations

The first and vital point to be borne in mind is that in homeopathy dosage is not related to body weight. The governing factors are the severity of the condition and the natural resilience of the patient. This means that animals of widely differing body weights will receive the same number of tablets (pillules, etc.) at any one administration. One implication of this, in the farm situation, is that weight variations between individual animals need not be considered. Also, as already discussed in Chapter 3, no matter what the physical size of the dose given at any one time, the body will treat it as a single dose in energy terms. Thus one tablet or pillule will be as effective as six given at the same time. A combination of the *potency* of the remedy and the *frequency* of its administration makes up the dosage, and it was shown in Chapter 3 that the higher the potency, expressed as a dilution, the greater the healing potential. The more accurate the prescription, the more does this apply. The other consideration is the strength of the patient's vital force. This of course is not an absolute but is a matter of clinical judgement in each case.

The underlying aim is to match the energy of the illness with an equal healing energy.

In acute disease in an otherwise healthy animal, there is often a high-energy output as a result of a strong challenge to the body and a strong response to that challenge. The reaction of the body is an indication that the vital force is robust, and can therefore respond to a vigorous stimulation. The homeopathic dosage will reflect the energetic situation by employing a high potency administered frequently. Thus an acute trauma in an otherwise healthy animal may be treated using Arnica at a potency of M administered every 5–10 minutes. An acute infection with a temperature of 105°F (40°C) may call for Belladona in similar dosage as opposed to a lower potency of 30c at the same frequency, which latter would not give a strong enough healing energy to oppose the illness. If the 30c were employed then an increased frequency of administration would be necessary to achieve the same energy input.

In the above examples, the body will receive a strong healing stimulus frequently.

However, in cases where the vital force is weakened, either by pre-existing disease (e.g. renal failure) or because the patient is succumbing to the disease, such a regime can be counterproductive. Here the frequency of administration may remain the same but the potency will be reduced, possibly to levels of 6c. The body will receive milder healing stimuli to which it can respond, while the frequency of the stimulation ensures that the healing process is continuous.

In chronic conditions, where it is necessary to reverse a lower grade but deeper-seated imbalance, when using the decimal or centesimal scales, the frequency of administration will be reduced, but the potency may be increased. With the LM potencies, their different method of preparation enables them to be used on a much more regular and long-term basis, starting with the lowest (LM1) potency and rising through the scale as appropriate. The factors affecting the choice of potency are discussed below. In energetic terms the essence of these situations is that the whole interplay of challenge and response is more muted, and there is involvement over a wider range of organs. Also, the basic fault is that there is an inability of the body to reverse the 'dis-ease' process. This may be due to suppression as was discussed in Chapter 4, or to an inherently weak vital force. Indeed, continuous suppressive treatment will in time lead to a weakening of the vital force. Thus dosage must reflect the requirement of a potency that will stimulate but not overwhelm the vital force, while at the same time pushing the healing process forward. It is often necessary to proceed stage by stage, clearing each layer in accordance with Hering's law (page 43), and allowing the body time to cure itself at each level. In practice this means a low frequency of administration, allowing the action of one dose to work itself out before repeating or changing remedies. This results in the administration of remedies at intervals measured in weeks or months.

The acute flare-up in the course of a chronic disease falls between the two extremes discussed above. While the acute element in the situation calls for more frequent administration, the weakened state of the patient militates against over-vigorous treatment. In these cases the frequency is most likely to resemble the conventional pattern of night-and-morning or thrice-daily administration.

This convergence is of course purely coincidental. It will already be apparent that the rationale of dosage regimes in the conventional and homeopathic disciplines is entirely different. Another major difference between the two systems is that whereas in the conventional world a full course of treatment is given even if there is clinical resolution before its end, in homeopathy treatment is stopped as soon as there is an improvement, and it is not restarted as long as that improvement continues. If there is complete resolution of the problem with one dose, that is all that needs to be given. If improvement ceases before there is complete recovery, or there is any regression, then the remedy is repeated. Even if several doses were given initially, a single dose may be all that is required to move the case forward again. Rather than the administration of a single unit of the remedy, the so-called 'single divided dose' is often used. This is classically the administration of three units at 12-hour intervals over a 24-hour period; sometimes the alternative of one dose daily for three days is used.

The point to remember is that homeopathy is concerned with setting a natural healing reaction going and, if necessary, boosting it and keeping it going until complete cure is attained. On the farm, where detailed assessment of the response of individual animals may be difficult, a course of treatment of set length is usually selected, but the emphasis is on its being of short rather than long duration (4–5 days).

The choice of route of administration depends on the species being treated and the exact nature of the problem. The prime consideration is to facilitate the absorption of the remedy's energy through a clean mucous surface. The mouth is the most common surface employed with the remedy being dissolved by the saliva. The nasal and vaginal surfaces can also prove useful, with remedies being administered via sprays, or by using the medium of the drinking water. With herds and flocks these latter may be the only practical means. The frequency of administration in these situations will depend primarily on the factors discussed above, but management considerations may dictate some compromises.

Potency Considerations

In general terms, to select the right remedy is more important than to select the right potency. The wrong remedy will be of no benefit whilst the correct remedy in a lower than ideal potency will still have some effect, and the dosage of the correct remedy can be adjusted by altering either the potency or the frequency of administration. That is not to say that potency is unimportant, but it is secondary to remedy selection.

It has been established that the higher the potency, the greater the potential for curative action. At the same time, the higher the potency, the less margin for error there is in remedy selection. The range of action of a remedy is in *inverse* proportion to its potency – that is, a low potency will have a more superficial action on a wider range of symptoms, while its depth of action has a more *direct* proportion to the potency. (It must be remembered that potency scales are not linear.) A high potency of the correct remedy will hit hard and fast at the root of the problem. A low potency of the correct remedy will have some beneficial effect but it is unlikely to be strong enough to bring about a cure. A high potency of the wrong remedy will have no effect. Even if the remedy selected is similar to the correct one, in high potency its powerful action will be on too narrow a front to affect the centre of the disease. On the other hand, a low potency of such a related remedy will overlap the simillimum picture to some extent and will therefore have some healing effect. The situation is analogous to the use of a blunderbuss as opposed to a high-precision rifle.

A basic rule of potency selection is therefore 'the more certain the prescriber is of the correct remedy, the higher the potency that can be employed'. Confidence in remedy selection can only be achieved by consideration of the higher levels of symptoms in the hierarchy. Good mental and general symptoms are essential. Prescriptions based largely on local symptoms should be given in low or medium potency.

There are however other factors that influence potency selection. The energy dynamics of the disease process as outlined above are important. An advanced pathology is often indicative of a weakened vital force, and hence a lower potency should be used. Conversely, pathologies such as malignancies may have a high local energy but the potency being used for their treatment should still be kept low to moderate, as the risks of over-stimulation are too great. The level at which the effect is desired must be borne in mind. If the prescription is aimed at a local level then the potency used will usually be lower. Even in the case of a correct remedy a high potency may fail to have an effect on a local lesion. A desired effect at a deeper or behavioural level will, all other things being equal, indicate a higher potency.

A high potency will give depth of action, getting to the heart of the case and producing a basic change in the function of the whole system, while a low potency will give breadth of action, with a more superficial effect on a range of symptoms. Where flocks or herds are being treated as a whole, a medium potency (30c) is usually the most practical.

A type of preparation occasionally used is the 'potency chord', a concept developed in the second half of the 20th century. In this the same remedy at different potencies is given in the same dose. The result is thought to resemble that of a musical chord, thereby producing a greater resonance with the disease process. The effect is not the same as giving the remedy in separate doses of ascending potency. It is not widely used although its proponents claim good results, especially in chronic disease.

When smaller animals such as hamsters, guinea pigs or birds are being treated there is a general tendency to need higher potencies to achieve the same response. This is a function of the higher metabolic rate of these species, whereby the energy of the remedies is consumed more quickly, irrespective of the disease. There are some remedies that change their effect according to the potency that is administered. Hepar Sulph. and Mercurius both encourage suppuration in low potency but abort it in high. Fortunately for the memories of homeopaths, these are the exception rather than the rule!

Different homeopathic traditions will have slightly different ideas as to what constitutes a low, medium or high potency, but as a general rule it may be considered that up to 12c is a low potency, between 12c and 30c a medium one, and above 30c a high one. The decimal scale follows the equivalent divisions but the LM scale does not follow the same rule. Treatment using the LM potencies does not involve the same considerations of 'low' or 'high', with courses being generally begun at the LM1 level and rising from there if necessary in a steadily ascending pattern.

Various advantages are claimed for the LM potencies. One is that there is a reduced risk of aggravations and untoward reactions, even with long-term usage. That does not mean, however, that reactions are never seen whilst using the scale. Another claimed advantage is that they are able to obtain better results with less upsets in cases where there has been much previous conventional medication, and hence potentially much suppression. Finally, in cases where there is much advanced pathology their use is widely considered to be safer and more effective than with the other scales.

Remedies made from healthy glandular tissues (sarcodes) can be used to either stimulate or inhibit the action of the appropriate gland in the patient, and the potency is selected according to the physiological effect that is required. In this *particular* context, the change from low to high potency is different to that given above, and occurs at the 7c point. Low potencies of below 7c should be given if stimulation of the gland is required, while those over 7c are needed for reduction of activity.

Using a remedy in ascending potencies is often a means of keeping a healing process moving forward, although there are occasional situations where a reduction of potency will re-start a stalled process. This is probably linked to the reactive potential of the vital force. However, there are some remedies, notably Conium, where its use in steadily ascending potencies enhances its effect. Using a remedy in ascending potencies may also be applicable in cases where it is necessary to gradually restore an intrinsically high vitality that has received a temporarily debilitating challenge, for example in a dog collapsed with parvovirus.

Interpreting the Response

The first consideration is when to assess the situation following the administration of a remedy. Acute cases require rapid responses that will vary from a few minutes in the case of an acute anaphylactic shock to a few hours in less per-acute conditions. The response is clear-cut, with a return to normal activity or a significant improvement being clearly recognisable. If there is no response from the first few doses then another remedy should be selected. As a rule of thumb there should be a response within a maximum of four doses. While four doses of the wrong remedy will not cause any adverse effects, it must be remembered that the patient may deteriorate due, in effect, to not receiving any treatment.

In assessing the response to treatment, a knowledge of the normal course of the disease is important. In acute disease, the assessment of the response is made relatively soon after the administration of the remedy. In chronic disease the converse is true.

Homeopathy acts by stimulating the body's own responses – once stimulated, those responses must be allowed time to work themselves out. The dosage may be small, perhaps one single tablet, or three tablets given at 12-hour intervals (the so called 'single divided dose') but the assessment should not be made for at least two weeks in the absence of any reactions that worry the owner. It must also be realised that a reaction to treatment which concerns the owner may in fact be an encouraging development. The phenomenon of the therapeutic aggravation is always possible. This is an apparent worsening of all the presenting signs and symptoms, but it is in fact part of the healing effect and as such is, in general terms, to be welcomed. It is important to make clear to the owner the differences in interpretation between the conventional and homeopathic approaches.

Possible responses

In a chronic disease there are a number of possible responses. However, in cases coming to homeopathic treatment after receiving recent allopathic medication, another consideration must be borne in mind. In addition to those changes brought about by the remedy, there is always the possibility of changes appearing in the presenting picture as a result of the withdrawal or variation of dosage of the conventional drugs.

(i) *No change at all in any direction.* The likeliest cause is that the wrong remedy has been selected. In this event the case must be reviewed and a new remedy selected. Before accepting this interpretation, it is advisable to check with the owner as to their exact method of storage and administration of the remedy (Chapter 3). Owners can on occasion be very ingenious in devising dosing techniques, and some of these may interfere with the action of the remedy. If after doing this the same remedy is still strongly indicated, the possibility of a block to the response should be considered. This is usually some previous event in the animal's history – an infection, vaccination, mental trauma, routine medical or surgical intervention and so on. It must be remembered, when exploring this aspect of the case, that homeopathy considers things to be relevant which the conventional world dismisses as unconnected to the presenting problem. Similarly, ongoing preventive measures such as routine systemic flea treatment may adversely affect the body's ability to respond. If such a block is found then this must be removed, either by withdrawing the routine medication or with another remedy before returning to the first. Another possibility is that the remedy is correct but that the potency selected has been far too low. In this case there will have been some response but it will have been so slight as to be unnoticed.

(ii) *No physical change but a definite mental improvement.* This is an indication that things are moving in the right direction in accordance with Hering's law. The mental levels, being generally more important to a case than the physical, will respond first. The selected remedy should be continued with in the same potency but, before repeating, time must be allowed for the full action of the remedy to have worked through. The time required for this will vary with both the animal and the remedy, and although reference is made in the standard works to the length of action of remedies, these are only a general guide. The only sure assessment is by observation of the animal. However, if the choice of remedy has been made using mainly mental symptoms, a re-assessment of the case may be necessary in order to ensure that all aspects of the case have been covered.

(iii) *A steady improvement in all aspects of the case.* The correct remedy has been chosen and administered at the correct potency. Do not change the remedy. If improvement is still continuing, wait until it ceases before re-assessing the case. If the improvement ceases before there is complete cure, but is maintained, repeat the remedy at the same potency.

(iv) *An all-round improvement which ceases before cure and then regresses to some degree, or reverts to the original state.* The remedy is right but the potency is wrong. Repeat the remedy but change the potency. The required change will usually be upwards, although occasionally lowering the potency is necessary to take the case forward. There is, unfortunately, no easy way to predict this, and so in practice the initial change is always to increase the potency as this is by far the commonest requirement.

(v) *An initial worsening followed by a steady improvement.* Here the right remedy has been given but the potency has been too high, and a therapeutic aggravation (see below) has been produced. It is also possible in the early stages for there to be a worsening of the presenting symptoms accompanied by an improvement in the mental well-being of the patient. Because the mental aspect of a case takes precedence, do nothing for as long as the improvement continues. If the improvement ceases before complete cure, repeat the remedy in a lower potency.

(vi) *Considerable improvement but some symptoms remaining.* In this case wait until all improvement has ceased. The remedy is correct. Repeat if necessary.

(vii) *Improvement in presenting symptoms but re-appearance of previous symptoms.* This is Hering's Law in action. The remedy is correct. Wait and the re-emerging symptoms will usually pass without further treatment, with only support treatments for the welfare of the patient being necessary. For this, on some occasions, a new remedy may be required in the short-term.

(viii) *Some improvement but new symptoms appearing.* The remedy has brought out new symptoms of the case that were not apparent before. This may be because either previous medication was suppressing the symptoms, or the case initially presented with a narrow range of symptoms from only one aspect. These are what Hahnemann referred to as 'one-sided cases'. The action of the remedy has revealed a new layer of the disease and a new remedy must be selected that matches the new presenting picture.

(ix) *No change in the presenting symptoms, but the appearance of new symptoms which have not been there before.* This indicates a poor remedy selection. What are appearing are symptoms of the remedy, not the disease. The greater the number of new symptoms appearing, the worse the remedy selection. Review the case and select a new remedy.

It is important when gauging the response to a remedy to review all aspects of the case. As mentioned previously, owners tend to focus on the sign or symptom that is of most concern to them. In addition, they have often had experience of the effects of conventional treatment on their animals. Although these effects may have been suppressive, as far as the owner is concerned they have produced a rapid, and in many cases, complete removal of the presenting signs. The effect of homeopathic treatment is judged by them against this yardstick. Thus further questioning of an initial report of 'no change' may in fact reveal that there has been a significant amelioration or alteration in a number of aspects of the case.

It must also be realised that although the possibilities are stated in 'black and white', in the clinical situation we are often confronted by 'grey'. The basic rule is *if in doubt stop the remedy and wait.*

Clinical Provings

The concept of provings has already been met with in the context of ascertaining the range of activity of a remedy. It is however possible to produce a proving in a patient during treatment. In these cases, signs and symptoms present in the remedy picture, which are not part of the disease picture, are produced in the patient. There are two possible reasons for this.

The first is that the patient is particularly sensitive to the remedy. In these animals (and people) the lower potencies as well as the higher can produce the reaction. Because of the sensitivity there will also be a curative action. The best course of action is to wait, and in most cases the symptoms of both the proving and the disease will subside. If it is felt that because of the distress produced, something must be done, then the remedy should be antidoted (see below). A problem can arise if, having waited, the curative process is not complete, and it may be possible in this situation to use a similar remedy in low potency to take the case forward. If the original remedy is still strongly indicated, then the associated bowel nosode (Chapter 13) can be used.

The second reason for a clinical proving is the overuse of a remedy that has been successful in alleviating symptoms. This is one of the problems which can occur due to the easy availability of homeopathic remedies, albeit in the lower potencies. If Rhus Tox. has been prescribed with success for an arthritic condition, the owner may decide that, as one tablet night and morning for a week has produced such a good improvement, then one tablet three times a day indefinitely will produce a better one! In due course the animal presents with an irritant skin rash which is part of the total Rhus Tox. picture, but nothing to do with the original presenting complaint. At the same time the original complaint may well have worsened again. Farmers may overuse remedies in an attempt to control ongoing conditions such as mastitis, and end up exacerbating the problem. Inexperienced veterinary surgeons may also fall into the same trap, not necessarily by increasing the dose but by continuing with the remedy for too long. The first thing to do is to stop the remedy. After that, wait and the situation will usually resolve itself quickly, because the continued overuse of the remedy is keeping the artificially created disease going, and once that stimulus is removed the body can return to its previous state (Chapter 4). If the reaction does continue it may, in occasional cases, be necessary to antidote its action.

Palliation

It is possible to palliate with homeopathy just as much as with conventional medicine, and in chronic conditions such as arthritis this may be all that can be done. Although the aim should always be to cure, in some cases – due to advanced pathology and/or the effects of previous medication in weakening the body's systems – it may be that palliation is all that is obtainable. From the welfare point of view this is desirable as, used properly, homeopathy can give the advantages of relief for the animal without the problems of side effects from conventional medication. However, it should always be borne in mind that what is being achieved is only palliation, and the consequences of this must be considered.

As discussed in Chapter 5, there is a difference of perception between homeopathy and conventional medicine over chronic disease and, for the orthodox mind, a tendency to accept the removal of symptoms as cure. In contrast, for the homeopath the diagnosis of 'arthritis' is not an entity in itself, but is only one aspect of a whole disease picture. By concentrating any type of treatment solely on the presenting local signs of that one aspect, all the rest of the disease process is being ignored, and may well worsen. A rush into palliation may well turn a curable case into an incurable one via a suppressive reaction.

Once the aim of palliation is, for whatever reason, accepted, a conventional style of dosage should not be assumed after an initial successful prescription and response. If it is, a clinical proving as outlined above may be produced. After the initial course, treatment should be stopped and only restarted when symptoms recur. It is not necessary to wait until the situation has fully deteriorated again, but merely until there are any signs of a relapse. It is important to keep a note of the time that has elapsed from the end of the initial course to the point when treatment is started again. Nor will it be necessary to repeat the whole of the first course, but only one or two doses should be required. Once control of the symptoms has been restored, then it is again necessary to wait and note the time interval until signs of worsening reappear, at which time one or two doses of the remedy are once more repeated. In this way it is possible to build up a picture of how frequently the remedy is genuinely needed, and if a consistent pattern emerges, then the onset of symptoms can be pre-empted by administering one dose the day before the expected deterioration. It may be that treatment is required daily, as the energy of the remedy is used up rapidly, but let the animal show that this is the case. In other cases the dosage required will be more intermittent, and there may be seasonal variations in the required dose. However, there will be no danger of a clinical proving if the animal has been allowed to indicate the dosage required.

Aggravation

Aggravation in homeopathic terms is not the undesirable occurrence that it is in the conventional world, and it is important to make owners aware of the big difference between the two systems. Conventionally, aggravation represents a genuine worsening of the condition, and this is particularly serious when it occurs in spite of treatment. In homeopathy, an aggravation will always follow correct treatment and as far as the prognosis is concerned it is very good news indeed. For this reason it is often referred to as a *therapeutic aggravation.*

Homeopathy works by stimulating the body to correct the imbalance inherent in the disease situation. The vital force acts, on the physical plane, through what is conventionally considered as the psychoneuro-endocrine system. The signs and symptoms on which the remedy selection is based are the outward manifestations of the body's attempt to cure itself. Thus an intensification of those manifestations as a result of treatment indicates an increase in the curative effort.

In reality there is an aggravation with every successful prescription, but in the best cases it is so mild that it passes unnoticed. Certainly, in veterinary work, the owner or handler is only likely to spot a severe aggravation. This usually occurs when the remedy is correct but the potency is too high and the stimulation of the vital force has been too vigorous. If the patient is particularly sensitive to the remedy an aggravation can occur with a low potency.

A common feature of an aggravation is that, in a physically orientated condition, although there will be a marked increase in the intensity of the physical signs, there will also be an improvement in the mental well-being of the patient. As would be expected, because the remedy is correct but is providing an overstimulation, an aggravation will occur very early in a course of treatment, usually after only one or two doses. As a rule of thumb, the sooner it occurs, the more excessive the potency. The most important action to take is to STOP THE TREATMENT AND WAIT. As it is an overstimulation of a desired effect, it will work its way out quickly, leaving the patient better in all respects. If the treatment is continued the reaction will be prolonged to pathological proportions.

Although an aggravation is to be welcomed in the vast majority of cases, there are a few instances where it can be harmful. These are where there is very advanced pathology. Care must be taken with cases of malignancy in this respect, and aggravations when treating epilepsy can have serious consequences. Potency considerations, as already discussed, become important in these situations.

There is one variation of the above which will be met with occasionally in chronic disease. This may be termed an *externalising aggravation.* Here there is a marked apparent worsening of the pre-senting symptoms on the skin in response to the remedy, plus the appearance of new lesions on other parts of the body. However, there will still be the improvement in general wellbeing that is found in other aggravations. This will usually occur in cases where there has been suppression of the full disease picture. Thus a condition that manifests as, for example, a chronic otitis externa under suppressive treatment, may, following the administration of a correct remedy, develop into a generalised skin condition. The appearance of this implies that the remedy was correct, and that its full picture in relation to the disease is appearing. It is also an indication that the reaction of the body is in accordance with Hering's Law, i.e. from inside to out. It is to be welcomed, but in these cases the subsequent resolution will be more prolonged than in the more usual acute therapeutic aggravation, and may well require the use of other local remedies as part of the case management.

Antidoting of Remedies

Various external factors may interfere with the action of remedies but in this context the antidote to a remedy means another homeopathic remedy, whose symptom picture is such as to oppose the first remedy picture. This, of course, implies a degree of similarity between the pictures, as one artificial disease is being replaced by another. Many claims are made in the materia medicas for such interactions, and some do undoubtedly exist, but others may be not as accurate. However, it is necessary to bear the possibility in mind.

Another aspect of the phenomenon is its deliberate use to counteract the induced proving or aggravation of a remedy. In general terms it is best wherever possible to allow these reactions to subside by themselves, but there may be occasions where it is necessary to intervene. The effect of the antidote may be complete or partial, but either will be sufficient to control the situation. A specific antidote for the triggering remedy may exist, but there are some that have a wide application in this regard. Nux Vomica, Camphor and Coffea are three such that are widely used, and of these Camphor has the widest application. The potency used should be moderate, with 30c being the standard, and the frequency should be 'short and sharp' – three doses in 24 hours (the single divided dose).

Another way of achieving the same result is to use the same remedy as has produced the reaction, but in much higher potency. This approach must be used with caution, and must *not* be employed in patients where the cause of the initial reaction is an intrinsic sensitivity.

The Second Prescription

The second prescription is not the second attempt to find the right remedy. It is the remedy chosen after the first one has had an effect. Its selection will be determined by the exact response of the first, and this must be carefully evaluated, as indicated above.

The response may well give a further indication of the inherent strength of the vital force. It may also not entail a change of remedy, only a change of potency. Rushing in to make a second prescription too soon is probably the commonest single fault in homeopathic prescribing. The virtues of *positive inactivity* cannot be overstated.

Once the healing reaction has been started in the body the presenting picture will begin to change, but the process can only progress at the speed of the body's own reactions, and this reactivity will vary between patients. Too early a reassessment of the case will mean that the new prescription is made on the basis of an incomplete body reaction, and hence on a symptom picture that is still changing. This will mean not only that the prescription will not be as accurate as it should be, but more seriously that the development of the whole case may be jeopardised.

Unicist Prescribing and Mixtures of Remedies

The plethora of prescribing methods found in homeopathy can be confusing for the newcomer, and in order to understand the claims of the various approaches it is necessary to consider the basic principles behind each.

Unicist prescribing follows the classic pattern as laid down by Hahnemann. With the later development by Kent of the concept of the constitutional remedy, the idea may be gained that homeopathy is about only giving one remedy. This is not so, and Hahnemann's instruction was to *only give one remedy at a time,* wait and assess its effect, and then move on. In fact in his later years he would at times change remedies with great frequency, but it was always one remedy at a time.

Since the advent of the constitutional concept, there has developed a style of prescribing involving the use of the constitutional remedy (Chapter 9) together with a more pathological prescription. This is in accordance with Hahnemann's ideas, as he also stated that different remedies might be the simillimum for different aspects of a case. The ultimate aim is always to address the totality of the case.

The practice of using mixtures of remedies is, however, different. The rationale is that a mixture of remedies that all have a known action on a particular organ or system (a) must have the required remedy in there, and (b) may produce a synergistic effect.

They are therefore essentially pathological prescriptions. Hahnemann opposed this approach in both the allopathic and homeopathic worlds on the grounds that there is no way of knowing what is doing what in the mixture, and that there could be antagonistic effects.

These mixtures, also sometimes referred to as complexes, are used widely in mainland Europe and to some extent in the UK and there is undoubtedly some effect from them. A major area of use is in acute disease, especially via over-the-counter sales direct to the public, and here they may well hasten resolution of the condition.

However, in chronic situations their effects are often at a palliative or suppressive level only. The reader is referred back to the section on palliation for an assessment of the effects of such on the total disease process, and the limitations of that approach in deep-seated chronic disease.

Many questions still remain unanswered concerning the rationale of using these mixtures of remedies in one preparation. The number of remedies involved may well be relevant, with an increasing question mark arising as the number exceeds three or four. The method of preparation of the mixture may also be relevant – does the potentisation take place using a mixture of the mother tinctures as a starting point, or are various separately prepared potencies just mixed together? The latter is probably the most common method. There is also the question of the combination of remedies at different potencies, which appears to some prescribers as an extremely questionable practice. Preparation in these cases must, of course, be by means of mixing pre-prepared potencies. According to accepted philosophy the body in these cases will react to the stronger artificial disease, that is the higher potency in the mixture, granted that there is a remedy match at some level. Yet it cannot be denied that some beneficial effects are often seen following the use of mixtures, and these cannot be ignored. The only way their use may be compatible with the tenets of classical homeopathy is if the mixtures are in fact acting in their own right as new remedies which have not yet been proved. Many established remedies, especially those of plant or animal origin, contain a number of substances that together combine to produce the clinical picture; for instance, Lycopodium contains both Alumina and Silica, which are established remedies in their own right with different remedy pictures.

Such mixtures are not the same as the 'group simillimum' discussed above. In the latter the choice of remedies is closely linked to the presenting disease picture, whereas the mixtures are produced from more general considerations and thus lack the individualisation that lies at the heart of the homeopathic method.

Reference

Handley, R. (1997). *In Search of the Later Hahnemann*. Beaconsfield: Beaconsfield Publishers.

Chapter 9

Constitutional Prescribing

The Concept of the Homeopathic Constitution

'This drug (Acid Nit.) acts more beneficially with patients of tense fibre (brunette) and less to those of lax fibre (blonde).' [Hahnemann, in *Chronic Diseases*]

As evidenced by the above quotation, Hahnemann himself noted that certain homeopathic remedies were more frequently indicated in particular types of patient, or patients of a certain 'constitution'. The concept of the homeopathic constitution therefore suggests that the mental, general and physical characteristics of a patient in health may be of value in selecting a suitable homeopathic remedy for that patient when suffering from disease. The corollary to this is that patients of certain mental and general characteristics may suffer from similar physical symptoms when ill; indeed, it may be possible to predict from these characteristics which physical symptoms the patient may develop when ill. Thus an animal which is fat, sluggish, seeks heat, and has a craving for eggs is likely to develop joint degeneration causing stiffness and pain which is worse in cold damp weather and better for exercise.

In relationship to this, consider two Labrador retrievers, both suffering from osteoarthrosis. Both have exostoses of the joints, and show symptoms of stiffness which are worse in cold and damp weather and better for movement. However, one is overweight, lacks energy and actively seeks heat, the other is slim, lively and dislikes heat. The former would require Calcarea Carbonica, the latter Calcarea Fluorica. The significant factor in making these prescriptions is that the symptoms of disease alone would not be sufficient to distinguish between the remedies; it is the characteristics of the animals when well which lead the veterinary surgeon to the correct remedy.

This is the essence of constitutional prescribing; the premise that the general characteristics of the patient when well can aid in determining the correct homeopathic remedy when the patient is ill.

The question then arises as to whether the constitution can change

104

over an animal's lifetime; the answer must be 'yes', as there is ample evidence for this. It is well recognised, for instance, that a young Pulsatilla type can develop into a middle-aged Silica or Sepia type. In the former case, the shy, timid, yielding and thirsty Pulsatilla becomes chilly and stubborn, while still retaining the shyness; in the latter, she becomes chilly, thirsty, snappy and antisocial. Having said this, however, there are a few animals whose constitutional tendency seems to be so strong that it persists throughout their lifetime, requiring the same remedy whatever disease condition they may suffer from. A dog belonging to one of the authors (P.G.) responded to Arsenicum Album for a chronic skin disease, diarrhoea, chorea and age-related nocturnal restlessness at various times during his lifetime. This situation is rare, however, and it is far more common for an animal to require a succession of different homeopathic remedies over the period of its life. In addition it should be noted that a constitutional remedy may not always be indicated in every case of disease. Certainly, in chronic disease, there will have been adequate time for the constitutional tendency to evidence itself, and a prescription on this level is likely to be essential at some stage of the treatment; however, a dog exhibiting constitutional traits of Calc. Carb. can still suffer from an acute gastritis which requires Arsenicum Album, and if hit by a car will still require Arnica. One may argue as to whether the constitution has been temporarily changed into that remedy state or whether the acute symptomatology simply overlies the constitutional tendency, but the fact remains that the practice of constitutional prescribing is largely confined to the sphere of the treatment of chronic disease.

The Advantages of Using the Constitutional Approach

Prescribing at the constitutional level has a number of advantages over other approaches:

(i) Using the constitutional approach adds enormously to the information on which to base a prescription; in the field of veterinary homeopathy, where so much information may be lacking in comparison to the human situation, this can be crucial. For instance, the rubrics appertaining to character of pain are largely unavailable for use by the veterinary homeopath, and delusions and dreams are similarly inaccessible. The totality of symptoms obtainable from an animal may therefore be considerably more restricted than that which a medical homeopath may have at his disposal. Being able to use the characteristics of the animal in health adds considerably to the body of information which comprises the homeopathic case, and therefore allows for a more far-reaching analysis than would otherwise be possible.

(ii) Prescriptions made on a constitutional basis are certainly capable of the most profound effects, as the remedies affect the patient at a most fundamental level.

(iii) Constitutional prescribing can offer a simple but effective means of rapid prescribing, and some of the greatest homeopaths, medical and veterinary, have been well on the way to making their prescriptions by the time the owner or patient has settled down in the consulting room, merely by noting the patient's physical appearance and demeanour.

It is important, however, not to get too obsessed with this concept; constitutional prescribing involves a certain amount of generalisation, and in a sphere of medicine where individualisation is the key to success, over-reliance on the patient's constitutional picture can lead to failure and inevitable frustration. Certainly the first prescription in a chronic case will often be made on a constitutional level, and the patient's history will contain important clues for this, but thereafter it would be wise to be more aware of the subsequent changes which the patient undergoes and to bias follow-up prescriptions towards these, rather than continue to rely too heavily on the patient's constitutional make-up.

Finding the Constitution by Repertorisation

As implied by the foregoing, identification of the constitutional remedy requires that information about the patient's characteristics be included in the selection of rubrics for repertorisation.

This adds enormously to the weight of information available for case analysis, and allows more scope to be selective in the choice of symptoms and therefore rubrics for repertorisation. It is here that the principles of the hierarchy of symptoms become of major importance. As constitution is largely defined by the mental and general symptoms, these take precedence over local symptoms. However 'strange, rare and peculiar' symptoms are of the highest grade of reliability and therefore of the greatest importance. Much debate ensues around how to select the precise rubrics for the analysis of a case but there are some general guidelines for selecting rubrics which are universally accepted.

(i) Not too large; the more remedies a rubric contains, the less useful it will be in individualising the patient. Ideally the rubric will contain 20–30 medicines, certainly no more than 100. However, it may at times be necessary use large rubrics if there is no alternative. Such an example would be 'Lack of vital heat', the rubric which represents a patient who seeks the warmth.

(ii) Not too small; rubrics containing one or two remedies only, especially if they are in plain type, may be incomplete and run the risk of inaccurately biasing the case analysis towards these medicines. These rubrics may however be useful as confirmatory information once a remedy has been selected.

(iii) Rubrics should contain a spread of grades of remedy (bold, italic and plain type, as explained in Chapter 7). These are more likely to help in separating similar remedies from each other in the analysis.

(iv) Choose rubrics which most precisely describe the symptoms observed. Especially when dealing with mental symptoms in animals, there may be a choice of rubrics which are only slightly different from each other. Careful consideration is necessary to ensure accuracy at this point.

(v) Choose rubrics which correspond to the symptoms which are most strongly and clearly exhibited.

(vi) Not too many rubrics. With computer programmes it is so easy to input rubrics that it is tempting to be less selective, but a few well chosen rubrics will produce far more accurate results than any number of less well chosen ones. Traditionally, around eight rubrics should cover the most important features of a case, but often three or four alone can convey the essence of the case quite adequately.

(vii) When weighting rubrics in a computer repertorisation programme, give more emphasis to those symptoms which are either exhibited most clearly in the patient, or are strange, rare or peculiar, and use the standard hierarchy of 'mentals before generals before locals'.

In this context, it is worth reiterating that repertorisation is most accurate when a few distinctive symptoms or characteristics, clearly exhibited in the patient, are accurately matched to medium-sized rubrics and, when using a computer repertory, the selected rubrics are precisely weighted before analysis is performed.

Using Constitutional Prescriptions

Inevitably the remedies used for constitutional prescriptions are nearly always taken from the major polychrests; the number of remedies recognised as such varies from homeopath to homeopath, but there are perhaps 30 or 40 commonly recognised constitutional pictures.

A prescription based on the constitution of the patient is capable of affecting the patient on a profound level; in consideration of this the most commonly-used dosing regime is comprised of a small number of doses of a high potency preparation administered over a short period of time. (The authors' preference is for three or four doses given at twelve-hourly intervals.) Sometimes the constitutional picture seems clear but the local symptoms are not covered by the constitutional medicine. In this case a high potency remedy may be prescribed on constitutional principles, followed by a low potency preparation aimed at the local symptoms. Some workers would advise giving the constitutional medicine alone in this case; others would hold that another medicine must exist which does cover both areas. Such is the debate which continues in the field of human and veterinary homeopathy on this rather contentious subject! Being so profound, the response to constitutional prescriptions can often be slow, and in an effort to gain more rapid improvement of the patient's condition some workers advocate the use of the same medicine at different potencies, either a high potency first, followed by a course of low potency medicine, or vice versa. Similarly, a 'multi-level' approach may consist of the use of organotropic medicines or specific nosodes alongside constitutional medicines.

As one delves into this fascinating area, one inevitably forms one's own conceptualisation of how homeopathic medicine affects the organism; in the meantime we would suggest that the concept of 'the constitution' be considered simply as the *tendency* of an individual bearing a particular pattern of mental and general characteristics towards the need for a particular homeopathic remedy – no more, no less.

Some Common Constitutional Pictures

Many generations of animal breeding have resulted in the selection of breed characteristics which often give a clue to an animal's constitution. This is especially true with dogs, where in any particular breed one constitution often predominates. This represents both a useful shortcut, and at the same time a rather dangerous trap. Certainly, breed characteristics are valid arbiters in deciding on an individual's constitution, but it should be understood that virtually any constitution may be represented in any one breed. Indeed, if an individual's characteristics run contrary to those normally expected in the breed, greater significance should be attached to them compared to those which are more commonly represented in the breed. Nevertheless certain breeds of any species are associated with particular homeopathic medicines and this can be of considerable use in assessing the constitution of an individual animal.

Arsenicum Album

Arsenicum is anxious and severely chilly. The Arsenicum dog enters the consulting room looking fearful and may panic when lifted onto the table. If carried, he clings to the owner and may struggle when approached by the vet. He is so frightened he may in fact snap, but this is simply from fear, especially the fear of being confined in a small space and unable to escape. At home he sits almost on top of the fire and will bask for hours in the midday sun. There is restlessness, especially after midnight; the twitchy old dog wanders about and will not settle, the horse with sweet itch paces the stable. This night-time aggravation is reflected in all the physical symptoms; gastroenteritis, asthma and atopy – all are worse after midnight, and even when apparently in good health the Arsenicum dog will occasionally get his owner out of bed to wander aimlessly around the garden for no apparent reason.

There is fastidiousness too; the racehorse keeps his stable in impeccable tidiness, piling up the droppings in one corner. The Arsenicum cat with renal failure still keeps herself pristinely clean and her litter tray in order, even going so far as to tidy the spilt litter into a neat little pile. The Arsenicum dog refuses to go through puddles or mud or otherwise soil his coat. If he does get dirty he spends ages meticulously grooming himself until he once again shines like new.

Arsenicum likes company; dogs dislike being left on their own and may bark or whine when left in the house; horses may get upset if their companions go off without them. There is also fear of enclosed spaces such as cages or cars, and the anxiety and restlessness so characteristic of this constitutional type may be triggered by such confinement. On the food and drinks side there is thirst for small quantities, and a liking for fruit and raw vegetables, in fact cold food of any kind. So chilly, anxious, restless and fastidious, a sipper of water and a lover of fruit and vegetables, such is Arsenicum.

Sulphur

Sulphur is hot and smelly. The fat, lazy dog, often with a history of chronic skin irritation greets the vet with a friendly wag of the tail and then slumps down on the cool floor and goes to sleep; standing is uncomfortable. Even when recently bathed they are smelly, and the coat always looks untidy. 'When I've groomed her she looks immaculate for ten minutes' is how one owner described her Sulphur bitch. In any case, Sulphur hates being bathed; they would much prefer to remain scruffy. Sulphur has redness and itching of the anus and passes foul-smelling wind. They hate the warmth; symptoms are aggravated by warmth and hence they always look for cool places – on the cold tiles of the kitchen floor, in the shade of a tree or in the draught by the door. The mucous membranes are dark red but beware of inspecting them, for Sulphur also has foul breath, even when the teeth and gums look clear. They are prone to diarrhoea, waking at 5 a.m. desperate to go out to pass a loose yellow stool.

Sulphur can also be lean and energetic, the boisterous 'life and soul of the party', but more often they laze around the house, looking for a cool draught to lie in and waiting philosophically for the next meal, whereupon they will eat anything put before them, sweet, salty or spicy – the favourite is the leftover curry which will be washed down with a long draught of cold water.

So generally a nice chap to have around, but Sulphur's noxious smell makes them less popular than might otherwise be the case, and don't expect a lot of moral support from the Sulphur animal; they are rather selfish creatures and are unlikely to take much notice of your problems as long as they are alright themselves.

Easygoing but self-centred, hot and smelly, with a love of spicy foods and a prodigious thirst; this is Sulphur.

Natrum Muriaticum

This remedy presents with apparent independence; 'apparent' because one of the key features of Natrum Mur. is the suppression of feelings, particularly of grief. It is often considered to be 'the cat's remedy' because it is perhaps the most common constitutional picture to present in cats. It is the cat who really does not seem to want company; he will always be found by himself, stuck away in a cupboard or out in the shed, only coming for attention when he wants it. Attempts at stroking or picking him up will either be resisted, or tolerated for a short time only, and the contact may be terminated with a bite or a scratch that says 'That's enough'. However, Natrum Mur. may become very attached to a single animal or person, and this is one of the characteristics which make the type so vulnerable to grief. The loss of an animal or human companion (and let us not forget the enormous emotional stress placed on an animal when it is rehomed) can send this animal into severe depression. The child's pony, sold on because its rider has 'outgrown' it, exhibits the Natrum Mur. constitution by sulking in the corner of the stable, avoiding eye contact, and kicking out when approached.

Conversely, the grief may be so well covered up that it is not apparent, and only when physical symptoms such as dermatitis appear can it be identified in retrospect. Natrum Mur. will also sulk; put her in kennels and she will make sure you feel guilty by ignoring you for days afterwards! Natrum Mur. is thirsty; not the dainty sips of Arsenicum but long draughts at long intervals. Heat modalities can be confusing; either chilly or hot, and although human Natrum Mur. avoids the sun this is not always the case in animals. Perhaps most commonly, the animal seeks heat indoors, but also loves to be out in the cool air. The animal is generally thin, despite a good appetite, though sometimes there is a bloated appearance as if too much fluid is retained; there is craving for salty foods such as potato crisps, and for fish. Most of all Natrum Mur. doesn't like its space invaded and in canine terms this means holding eye contact; look Natrum Mur. in the eye and they will avert their gaze; get too close physically and they may snap – just a warning, but enough to leave one in no doubt that this animal prefers to be alone. The desire for privacy extends to urinary habits and the Natrum Mur. animal will rarely micturate while anyone is watching; occasionally this extends to defaecation also.

So Natrum Mur. is independent, thirsty and thin, with a love of salty foods.

Calcarea Carbonica

The Calc. Carb. dog enters the waiting room slowly. After greeting the veterinary surgeon he slumps down in the corner and doesn't move for the rest of the consultation. Usually heavily built and often obese, with a large broad head, he is open and friendly but may be also a little timid.

He is chilly; he hugs the fire in winter and can be almost impossible to dislodge. If it is cold and wet he has no desire to go out; even at the best of times he prefers to stay in bed, and when eventually persuaded to take his morning walk may be so reluctant as to be just 'not worth the bother'.

However Calc. Carb.'s friendliness, coupled with his inner fear of the loss of his security, mean that he can indeed enjoy exercise, though his bulk and low energy level generally mean he is not the sort of dog who will run or even plod all day with any ease. His poor circulation cause him to be rather intolerant of hot weather and Calc. Carb. may find exercise hard work when it is warm, though he will always love a swim. Rarely any trouble, he is open and friendly with other dogs and loves people, even burglars.

Calc. Carb.'s appetite is prodigious; he will eat almost anything edible and lots that isn't, such as plaster off the wall or coal out of the scuttle. He may crave dry foods such as bread. With a 'cast-iron' digestive system he rarely has an upset stomach, though milk can occasionally aggravate and he may have a tendency to constipation. Paradoxically he may actually feel better in himself when he is constipated.

If he does have diarrhoea the stools may look like clay and he may pass a stool which starts off solid and then goes loose.

So Calc. Carb. is open, friendly, great with the kids and just the perfect family dog. But given the opportunity he will devour the contents of the rubbish bin and will be of little use as a guard dog. The Calc. Carb. cow is the big-boned Friesian who plods along at the back of the herd. She is obstinate but *not* aggressive and has a prodigious milk yield.

Phosphorus

Phosphorus bursts into the waiting room full of energy, jumps all over the vet and licks him. She is thin and deep-chested, often with a long nose and may well be red or liver in colour. She loves people and other dogs and just can't get enough attention, but may also be fearful, so much so that she may appear aggressive, barking at other dogs especially when on the lead.

The Phosphorus cat investigates the consulting room thoroughly before jumping on the vet's or the owner's lap and face-rubbing or wrapping himself around someone's legs. Many Phosphorus cats are ginger.

Phosphorus loves company, so if left alone the Phosphorus dog may bark or howl or be destructive, chewing up carpets, shoes or furniture. The Phosphorus cow panics when left alone in the collecting yard. She is bright in the eye, has long silky lashes and often a coat to match.

She is sensitive; to noise, to emotions and to changes in atmosphere, so much so that the approach of a thunderstorm may see her anxiously seeking the consolation of the owner. She may howl at doorbells or at the sound of a whistle or recorder. Phosphorus may appear to be clairvoyant, predicting when her owner will arrive home even when the timing is irregular.

Phosphorus may be chilly but may also find the heat of the fire or the sun intolerable and look for the cool of the kitchen floor or the shade of a tree.

The appetite is good, desiring salty foods and fish in particular. However despite the good appetite, she will rarely put on weight.

There is thirst for large quantities of cold water, which may be evidenced by preferring to drink from puddles, ponds and water taps rather than the water bowl.

Phosphorus then is bright, full of energy, loves attention and is playful to the extreme, but at the same time sensitive and fearful.

Pulsatilla

Pulsatilla is soft, gentle, mild and yielding. Most frequently Pulsatilla is female, but this does not preclude its use in males where the characteristics indicate it. The Pulsatilla bitch would love to be friendly but is a little too timid so instead she gently clings to the owner and stares lovingly at her. If she's too big to be carried, when approached she rolls over on her back in submission and may pass urine. Alternatively she will shrink away, but once she is persuaded that she is among friends she will thoroughly enjoy the attention and revel in the contact. She has a tendency to put weight on easily so appears plump and cuddly.

Pulsatilla likes gentle heat; in winter she will lie in front of the fire and will seek out the sunshine coming through the window or in the conservatory. However, she craves fresh air and will become overheated in a stuffy room; thereupon she will seek out the cool draught by the window or the door. In hot sunshine she will be found outdoors but sheltered from the sun in the shrubbery or under the garden seat.

Even in hot weather Pulsatilla will drink very little and her appetite can be capricious, sometimes going more than a day between meals. She loves cold foods and will happily chew ice and eat ice cream, though the latter may upset her stomach, as do all rich foods, especially fats.

Like Phosphorus, Pulsatilla, too, dislikes being left alone and may be destructive, but in a far less spectacular way than Phosphorus. She will sulk, too, but the changeability inherent in the Pulsatilla picture means that it is short-lived and as quickly as she became sullen, so too can Pulsatilla return to being bright and cheerful. Pulsatilla loves company; she feels insecure on her own, so will follow her beloved owner like a shadow, wherever she may go in the house; given the chance she will sleep on the owner's bed, or in the comfort of the armchair.

Pulsatilla makes a wonderful mother, so much so that she is prone to phantom pregnancies where she will make a nest, take toys to bed and produce large quantities of milk. Pulsatilla cows are welcome members of a dairy herd.

So Pulsatilla is timid, soft, gentle and yielding, loves affection, has little thirst but a digestive system which is sensitive to rich foods.

Lycopodium Clavatum

The essence of Lycopodium is lack of self-confidence, though this may not be immediately apparent, as the animal exhibiting this constitution attempts to cover up the insecurity by appearing aggressive and self-assured, especially if the challenge comes from an animal or human who is perceived to be weaker or in some other way inferior. The Lycopodium German Shepherd dog will bully bitches and smaller dogs, but acts submissively when challenged by a stronger male. In the household he will do all he can to dominate his owner but once the order is established he will be extremely obedient. Lycopodium is highly intelligent and will respond to training very quickly. He has a strong sense of duty, and hence will make a good guard dog, especially as he will bark ferociously at the door, even if his response is less than brave once the visitor is admitted.

The weak points of Lycopodium are the liver, intestines and urinary system. They virtually always show some disturbance of one of these areas, suffering from intermittent loose stools, wind and gastric problems on the one hand, or recurring cystitis, with or without urinary calculi on the other. The poor function of the liver is reflected in poor weight gains in young animals, and an inability to get moving in the mornings, when Lycopodium can be ill-tempered and difficult to get out of his bed. Conversely there is a general amelioration after midnight, which is almost pathognomonic of the remedy (Lycopodium is the only remedy in the rubric 'Midnight after; ameliorated' and is in bold type). Classically there is an aggravation between four and eight p.m.

Appetite is often poor, eating is often followed by bloating; the animal eats a few mouthfuls and walks away, returning later for more. There is a strong desire for sweet foods.

The sluggish circulation of Lycopodium means that the animal is basically chilly, but at the same time may be easily overheated and seek cool air and cool surfaces to lie on.

Lycopodium is therefore cowardly, but if threatened can turn nasty. He is thin, full of gas, and prone to urinary problems or digestive upsets such as colic.

Note: A constitutional type can be exhibited by a member of either gender. In the interests of the narrative, the foregoing descriptions are generally confined to male or female, but this should not be taken as indicating that the type is only represented by animals of that gender.

Chapter 10

Obstacles to Cure

Reference to Paragraph 3 of the *Organon*, as quoted on page 4, will reveal Hahnemann's observation that for homeopathic medicine to exert its effect, any obstacles to cure must be removed. This is a basic principle of any form of medicine, but in consequence of the energetic nature of homeopathy, the obstacles may be rather different from those one might consider in conventional medicine.

Structural

This term is used to encompass all those physical conditions which can prevent a homeopathic remedy (or indeed any form of medical therapy) from exerting a beneficial effect to the maximum of its potential. Obviously an injured limb must be rested, and a fractured long bone may require surgical fixation; poorly-fitting harnesses and collars must be removed and ingrowing toenails clipped. Overgrown hooves must be trimmed and ill-fitting saddles replaced. However, consideration must also be given to poor conformation, and in a world of animal ownership where genetic abnormalities have been deliberately selected over generations, there will inevitably be limits to what can be achieved by homeopathy in treating the consequences. Then there are the consequences of poor management, such as heavily tartared teeth. While it is the authors' invariable experience that dogs and cats fed exclusively on raw foods never need their teeth descaling, if a patient is presented in a state of severe periodontal disease induced by poor dental hygiene, it may be essential to deal with this surgically before attempting any homeopathic treatment at all, particularly in view of the well documented general effects of such disease.

Perhaps this category may also include the working patterns of the patient; a dog engaged in agility training or sheep herding, or a horse involved in 3-day-eventing, will require cessation of those activities before any improvement of its locomotor problems can be expected.

Diet

Hahnemann's observation, quite revolutionary in its time, was that such factors as poor diet and damp living conditions were so important as to prevent the return to health which could otherwise be instigated by homeopathy.

It is certainly the opinion of the authors that poor diet is a major obstacle to cure in domestic animals, but the definition of poor diet may be somewhat at variance with received opinion.

Put simply, in any species, reliance on commercial, preserved diets will reduce the effectiveness of homeopathic treatment and in certain circumstances may block it completely. In small animals, several workers have proposed the benefits of fresh food diets, notably Billinghurst and Lonsdale, two Australian veterinary surgeons researching independently but both coming to the same conclusion, which is that dogs and cats have an innate dietary requirement for raw food, and particularly for raw bone. This can patently not be provided by any processed food. Indeed there are many reasons for the need for raw foods, one example being the requirement for polyunsaturated oils, obtained in the wild by the ingestion of herbivores' stomach contents. Billinghurst's book *Give Your Dog a Bone* (1993) provides a way of feeding dogs which can be simply followed, and the authors' experience in recommending this diet over ten years attests to its efficacy. The basis of this way of feeding, often referred to as the 'BARF' (bones and raw foods) diet, is the incorporation of a high proportion (up to 60%) of raw meaty bones in the diet.

Tom Lonsdale came at the subject from an interest in veterinary dentistry: he was not content with accepting the high incidence of periodontal disease universally recognised in domestic dogs and cats, particularly in the face of the effects of such disease on general health. It seemed obvious to him that this incidence was related to the widespread introduction of canned and dried 'complete' foods.

Lonsdale's views have not been universally accepted by the profession, but one result of his challenges was that in 1993 a literature review was undertaken by Professor David Watson of the Department of Veterinary Clinical Sciences, University of Sydney. His conclusion was that 'there is reasonable evidence that soft diets are associated with increased frequency and severity of periodontal disease'. The Australian Veterinary Dental Association now recommends bones be given two to three times a week for dental hygiene. It should be noted that, in this context, the authors consider that *any* processed food, be it canned or dried, should be regarded as 'soft'. For these reasons the authors support this particular system of feeding dogs, and other similar philosophies.

It is outside the scope of this book to go into detail about the feeding of small animals, but there is no doubt that feeding regimes consisting of total reliance on commercial 'complete' foods constitutes a major obstacle to cure. A similar challenge is presented by the increasing reliance by the horse owner on branded, processed feeds, and when the situation facing farm animals is considered, where production is boosted by the use of concentrated foodstuffs quite unsuitable to the ruminant digestive system, it becomes obvious that diet may well become a significant limiting factor to the response to homeopathy.

Having said all this, it is not always possible, and occasionally it is not advisable, to change an animal's diet completely; in the case of farm animals there are economic factors to take into account; with other species there may be unwillingness on the owner's part to put in the extra effort required in preparing a more natural diet; some animals may resist the change; yet others may be intolerant of one or more component. However, *any* move away from processed foods and towards foods which are presented in their natural state will be beneficial and is to be encouraged. Moreover, the most important point is that the veterinary surgeon should be aware of these issues and of the effect that poor diet may have on the effectiveness of homeopathic therapy.

Environment

It is universally recognised that certain diseases may be caused or at least exacerbated by certain environmental conditions. Respiratory disease caused by housing animals in overcrowded and poorly ventilated conditions (or in an animal whose owner smokes heavily), and the aggravation of arthritic pain in patients kept in damp conditions are two obvious examples. It is therefore essential that such factors are taken into account when treating animals homeopathically.

The environment may, however, be interpreted rather more broadly than simply in terms of the physical; mental and emotional wellbeing must also be considered. The response to homeopathy in cases of behavioural problems will be less than satisfactory if attention is not paid to the emotional atmosphere in which the patient lives. One of the authors (P.G.) rescued a Cavalier King Charles spaniel which was defaecating in the house; the problem resolved immediately on rehoming. In this field it is strongly advised that expertise is acquired or sought in becoming aware of the normal behaviour and social organisation within a particular species. This makes it much easier to understand what emotions an animal may be experiencing when challenged in this way. The correction of inappropriate training or management regimes may be an essential element in the homeopathic treatment of a behavioural problem. More importantly, the holistic view of disease which homeopathy engenders implies that the majority, if not all, of disease has a mental and emotional aspect, and the initiating cause is frequently of this nature. If the precipitating emotional stress is not addressed then homeopathy will be certainly less effective and may fail to resolve anything at all.

Orthodox Medication

There is little doubt that most orthodox drugs impede the action of homeopathic remedies. This is not surprising when one considers that the action of most of these medicines is in direct contradiction to that of homeopathy; anything which suppresses a reaction of the body will act counter to homeopathy, and considering the subtle energetic nature of homeopathic medicine it is only logical that such powerful drugs as corticosteroids and NSAIDs will antidote its effects. There is more debate about the effect of antibiotics; some workers consider that in certain circumstances antibiotics and homeopathy may work synergistically; others assert that the disruption to the bowel flora which ensues from a course of antibiotics renders the patient unable to respond adequately to homeopathy, and there are techniques in homeopathic therapeutics to deal with this. It is the authors' experience that short courses of antibiotics, perhaps given to deal with an acute infection or flare-up of chronic disease, do not seem to interfere markedly with homeopathic treatment; on the other hand, long courses of high dose antibiotics do seem to be suppressive and can seriously impair response to homeopathy.

Even replacement therapy of deficiency disease may present problems for the veterinary homeopath, and the authors have noted that patients who are receiving thyroid hormone or its analogues do not always respond as well to homeopathic medicines.

Perhaps the most important issue here is to be aware that *any* orthodox medication *may* interfere with the action of a homeopathic remedy and to take account of this in prescribing these medicines. Ideally, all orthodox medication should be stopped prior to commencing treatment with homeopathy, but this is frequently not possible, as exemplified by the atopic animal receiving long-term corticosteroid therapy. In such cases it is recommended that the orthodox therapy is reduced gradually. Firstly this may be possible as the homeopathic medicine starts to take effect, and secondly the reduction in dosage of the orthodox medicine will allow the homeopathic medicine to increase in its effect.

Similarly if there is an obvious 'Never Well Since' factor alluding to the administration of a conventional medicine, this may have to be addressed, for instance by administering a homeopathic potency of the medicine, before any other homeopathic remedy will take effect.

Finally it must be said that despite the forgoing, homeopathy does at times seem capable of acting despite heavy orthodox medication. It should never be rejected as being unsuitable merely because an animal has become dependent on conventional drugs.

Vaccination

Over-vaccination can be such a serious obstacle to cure that in this work the subject is afforded its own chapter.

It is only necessary at this stage to state that the authors are firmly convinced of the deleterious effect of over-vaccination on the progress of an animal under homeopathic treatment, and routine advice is for clients not to continue with annual booster vaccinations if they wish to afford their animals the full benefits of homeopathy. Alternatives such as routine titre-testing and homeopathic nosodes are offered where appropriate. All these issues are discussed fully in Chapter 14.

Previous Infectious Disease

In the same way that vaccination can create an obstacle to cure, so may a specific disease. Where the symptoms have arisen directly from a specific viral disease, for instance, it may be necessary to treat with the specific nosode before the full effect of remedies prescribed on homeopathic (rather than isopathic (q.v.)) principles is observed. Once again, look for the 'NWS'.

Surgery

In homeopathy, it is the premise that any symptom is the result of the vital force attempting to express its imbalance. It follows that to remove the organ or area involved in this expression not only obliges the organism to find other avenues for the expression of the imbalance, but also renders the organism incomplete and therefore at a disadvantage. The removal of an animal's tonsils or anal glands, as two of the most common examples, will therefore have the effect of creating an obstacle to cure. This is particularly apparent in the case of the anal glands, and it is the authors' experience that dogs which have had this type of surgery performed do not respond well to homeopathic treatment of the skin disease which inevitably seems to follow. Why this should be is a moot point but the likely possibility is that these glands exert an excretory as well as a secretory function, and that blocking that function obliges the excretion of toxins through other portals such as the external ear or the skin generally. It is well accepted that dogs with impacted anal glands commonly suffer from an associated otitis externa and this may be another aspect of this relationship. Whatever the intricacies, removal of anal glands constitutes a serious obstacle to cure and is something to be avoided if at all possible.

Similar caution should be exerted with regard to surgical removal of any organ. There is an ongoing debate as to the appropriateness of routine neutering of dogs and cats in particular; some veterinary homeopaths consider that neutered animals require more prolonged courses of homeopathic medicine than those who are entire. Further consideration of this issue is presented in Chapter 11 but it may be useful at this point to consider the effects of such surgery on the vital force of an animal.

Miasmatic Influences

Hahnemann developed the miasmatic theory to explain his failure to elicit long-term cure of many of his patients, and certainly in veterinary homeopathy a strong miasmatic tendency may render the patient more refractory to treatment than might otherwise be expected. When a patient does not respond to remedies which seem to be well indicated, addressing this miasmatic aspect of their disease may well be necessary before homeopathic treatment can exert its full potential.

Obstacles to cure, then, may present in any of a number of ways and it behoves the veterinary homeopath to be aware of the diversity of factors which can inhibit or prevent the response of an animal to homeopathic medicine.

Such a subtle form of medicine requires a relatively clear field in which to exert its effect on the vital force, and time spent exploring the area of obstacles to cure is time well spent.

References

Billinghurst, I. (1993) *Give Your Dog a Bone.* Bathurst, Australia: Billinghurst.

Lonsdale, T. (2001) *Raw Meaty Bones: Promote Health.* Windsor, Australia: Rivetco.

Watson, A.D. (1994) Diet and periodontal disease in dogs and cats. *Australian Veterinary Journal* **71**(10), 313-318.

Chapter 11

Miasms and Their Role in Disease

Understanding and Using Miasms

One of the major obstacles to understanding the miasms is the terminology, and the first confusing term is 'miasm' itself. It comes from the Greek '*miasma*' meaning a pollution or stain. In an age before microscopes and germ theory, it was generally used to describe noxious influences that appeared to be linked to outbreaks of disease, and these influences would include what are now thought of as infectious agents. When the connection that Hahnemann apparently made to scabies and the venereal diseases is added to this, the erroneous impression has been created that the theory is primarily about infections.

However, whilst the idea of pollution, as being a fouling that can be removed, gives part of the picture, staining has implications of something that produces a more permanent change, and it is this aspect of the definition that more accurately reflects Hahnemann's basic idea.

The other thing that must be remembered is that Hahnemann was a product of his age, who thought and wrote within the clinical experience and terminology of his time, whilst also attempting to introduce new concepts. It is necessary to get behind the terminology and realise that in essence the miasms are functional concepts rather than physical entities in order to see the underlying value of his ideas.

Because the miasmatic theory was developed in order to explain the sometimes unexpected and disappointing responses to treatment that Hahnemann and his colleagues obtained, there has remained to some degree an aura of negativity around it. However, it is an essentially positive concept that successfully accounts for those unexpected responses, and its clinical application offers a viable approach to many intractable problems. By taking account of the miasmatic patterns that appear in a case, the selection of an appropriate remedy can be made easier. Also, by following the changes in symptoms in relation to the miasmatic influences, it is possible to understand exactly what is happening as the body attempts to clear itself of disease, and hence plan a suitable case management strategy to assist its efforts.

Hahnemann's answer to the problem of chronic disease as outlined in Chapter 5 was the theory of miasms. As stated there he identified three of these which, for reasons that are discussed below, he named *psora, sycosis* and *syphilis*. The pollution or staining of an individual was described as being by direct contact in the case of psora and by coition in the case of the other two, which latter he linked to the venereal diseases gonorrhoea and syphilis. Psora was regarded as the most important agent. It was postulated as being capable of causing chronic disease in its own right, and Hahnemann considered that seven-eighths of all chronic disease was caused by this miasm. In addition, its presence was considered to be a prerequisite whenever sycosis or syphilis were implicated in the disease process. As also described in Chapter 5, the establishment of chronic disease in an organism was often considered to be the result of ineffectual or misdirected treatment of a more acute condition.

In one sense, defining the miasms is nothing more than a classification of types of body reactions that interact in situations of both health and disease. Grauvogl (1811–1877) was a German homeopath, who, working from his own perspective, also produced his own classification while taking account of the concept of miasms. Although his emphasis was towards the recognition of functional types in apparent health, whereas Hahnemann placed the function in the disease situation at the centre of his concept, there are nevertheless close similarities between these two views of body function.

Grauvogl postulated three types of constitution which were related to what he termed their 'biochemical state'. The different states were distinguished in part by their reactions to weather, and each was considered to produce different symptoms in disease.

He identified these as the carbonitrogenoid, characterised by slow metabolism and poor oxygen utilisation, the hydrogenoid with a strong affinity for and reaction to water, and the oxygenoid, linked to an accelerated metabolism of oxygen. He even went so far as to identify certain remedies as being most applicable to the treatment of his particular types. His classifications broadly equate respectively to Hahnemann's miasms of psora, sycosis and syphilis and the reason for the similarities is that both approaches are based on an interpretation of the basic physiological functions of the body. Whilst Grauvogl's ideas are similar in some ways to the homeopathic concept of constitution (Chapter 9), and Hahnemann's are more concerned with the function (or malfunction) of the body in the disease situation, both are based on the idea of the total physiological and psychological make-up of the patient providing the conditions in which disease can become established or maintained. Even Louis Pasteur (1822–1895), in spite of his involvement with the development of Germ Theory, finally came to acknowledge this concept, referring to it as the 'soil' in which disease can take root.

Although the development of the miasmatic theory resulted from experience in humans, and the terminology adopted was that of the human clinical situation, it must not be thought that the theory is any less applicable to animals. The ideas that are being expressed concern the basic dynamics of the living bodies in health and disease. Thus it is possible to recognise and treat a sycotic or syphilitic miasm in an animal even though it has never suffered from a venereal disease, and the psoric miasm may be present without a clinical case of mange.

The Basic Miasms

Psora

The name derives from the Greek word 'psora', which means an itch, or the 'itch disease'. In modern conventional practice this has come down to us as psoriasis. However, as a definition it can be misleading and the homeopathic concept of the miasm is much more profound. The root of the Greek word lies in the Hebrew word 'tsorat', which is defined as a groove, fault or pollution. It was a term applied to leprosy and the various other plagues that affected the ancient populations from time to time. The concept of a fault is much more what Hahnemann had in mind that merely pruritis – rather he viewed psora as an intrinsic weakness which manifested itself primarily in the skin, but which would, if denied that outlet, increasingly affect the deeper and more important organs. Its original external manifestation he identified as leprosy, which was, according to him, later modified into scabies as a result of improving hygiene and nutrition. (It should also be remembered that in Hahnemann's time there were not the accurate diagnostic aids that are enjoyed today, and so a diagnosis of scabies probably included a whole range of skin conditions rather than being the specific interpretation of the term currently employed.)

This historical connection that Hahnemann made has led to the misinterpretation that he regarded leprosy and scabies as manifestations of pure psora, whereas in fact he simply regarded them as the commonest and least harmful appearances of the miasm. In fact, it was the suppression of these external manifestations that he regarded as being at the root of the more serious and internal appearances of the disease state.

Because of his understanding of the basic nature of this miasm as a fault in the balanced response of the body, he maintained that it was impossible for either of the other two miasms to be clinically present in the body without the underlying presence of psora. His understanding of disease as essentially a functional upset, rather than a pathological entity, led him to state that psora was the miasm that was capable of causing the maximum of functional upset with the minimum of pathological change, and that it had the greatest potential of all for the derangement of the body's functioning. In modern parlance much of this would equate with a failure of homeostasis and normal function. It is this that produces the weakness associated with the miasm and allows the other two influences to establish themselves as clinical entities. Because of the role of the endocrine system in homeostasis, it is not surprising that may clinical conditions involving that system have a strong psoric element.

In all disease situations it is psora that produces the maximum of *functional* upset, whilst sycosis causes *increases* in discharges and tissue formation, and syphilis accounts for the greatest *physical destruction.*

Sycosis

This was linked by Hahnemann with gonorrhoea, although he makes it clear that the two are not synonymous. He also considered it to be the least important of the miasms, largely because gonorrhoea as a clinical entity was less serious than syphilis, and also because in his day it tended to appear as a major problem somewhat intermittently, usually linked to the close proximity of an army! Following its peak in the early years of the 19th century there was a steady decline in its incidence during Hahnemann's lifetime. The main features of the clinical disease are a copious discharge from the sheath in males, infection of and discharge from the cervix in the female, and the presence of the so-called figwarts – cauliflower-like warts that have a tendency to bleed easily. The infection is more common in males that females, but there are likely to be more serious consequences in the female.

The name of the miasm comes from the Greek word 'sykon', meaning a fig. As with psora, Hahnemann considered that the major factor in the creation of a clinical miasm was the inappropriate treatment of the material disease. In the 18th century there was considerable confusion and debate over whether there were two venereal diseases or only one. Hahnemann always considered that there were two, but others, notably the English surgeon John Hunter (1728–1793), took the opposite view. Thus systemic mercury was one of the standard treatments for all venereal disease and it was used in most cases, often in heroic doses. However mercury, whilst being a homeopathic and appropriate treatment for syphilis, is an unrelated (allopathic) and inappropriate one for gonorrhoea. There was also the widespread practice of removing the associated warts. This combination had the effect of influencing and suppressing only the superficial symptoms, whilst driving the underlying disease process inwards. This resulted in the production of more widespread manifestations of deep-seated disease in the body.

These manifestations were characterised by the excessive production of both tissues and discharges. The saying that 'gonorrhoea is the forerunner of catarrh' in many ways sums up the characteristics of the miasm, with its irritation of mucous surfaces and consequent discharges, its overproduction of new tissues and its general lay-down and production of pathological excesses in the body. Hahnemann's idea of its importance is probably no longer true today, and it may well have attained the position of being the most influential of the miasms. The most common clinical conditions seen today are not those of Hahnemann's time, with many of the major clinical entities that are now being encountered, such as cancer and irritable bowel syndrome, having a major sycotic component.

Syphilis

This is what Hahnemann described as 'the miasm of the venereal disease proper', reflecting the relative life-threatening properties of the two infections. It is the most destructive of both the associated clinical diseases and the miasms. In its primary state Hahnemann regarded it as an easily treated disease, and in *Chronic Diseases* states that 'there is on earth no chronic miasma, no chronic disease springing from a miasma, which is more curable and more easily curable than this'. However, if it is not properly addressed it will lead to the most serious of consequences. Tertiary syphilis is a fatal condition. In his time the treatment almost invariable involved the removal of the local chancre by external means, and this, as with the other conditions, had the effect of driving the disease process inwards.

The name derives from the Greek 'siphilos', meaning to cripple or maim, and this accurately describes the effects within the body of both the disease and the miasm. The latter may be thought of as nature's 'self-destruct button'. It is characterised by the physical destruction of tissues and the perversion of normal development. As with the other miasms, Hahnemann considered it to arise as a result of the suppression by inappropriate treatment of the clinical disease, but the full picture of the miasm is more than just the picture of tertiary syphilis.

Interpretations of the Theory

The original impression of the miasms as being solely the consequence of specific infections has been modified over the years, as it has been realised that Hahnemann himself never regarded them in such a simplistic light. The opening chapter of *Chronic Diseases* makes it clear that he considered the presenting picture of infection to be only 'some separate fragment of a more deep-seated original disease'. At one time a distinctly moralistic interpretation was introduced, notably by Kent and William Boericke, based on the original statements by Hahnemann concerning the role of coition in the establishment of two of the miasms. Both men were greatly influenced by the Swedish scientist turned theologian Emanuel Swedenborg (1688–1772) and the religious sect based on his teachings. According to them psora was equated with the original sin of the Judo-Christian traditions, whilst the acquiring of the sycotic and syphilitic miasms was associated with sexual impurity and promiscuous living.

Miasms are now broadly thought of as being a tendency in the individual to develop certain types of disease and to react to all challenges in a particular way. Current ideas are concerned with the way in which they affect the quality of what Pasteur described as the 'soil'. The exact miasmatic make-up of an individual is envisaged as arising partly from inheritance and partly from the influences of the challenges that have been met with during life. These two, grafted together, are considered as being capable of being passed on to the next generation in the absence of appropriate anti-miasmatic treatment.

The three basic miasms discussed above are those that Hahnemann identified, but there are nowadays concepts of other miasms. Both a cancer and a tubercular miasm have been described, and these can be recognised as established clinical entities, not only in cases of frank disease, but also in their behavioural and physiological patterns. Sankaran, with his own view of miasms, talks about other new patterns which he calls the malaria, ringworm, typhoid and leprosy miasms. His view of miasms is very much one of a progression through life, and in his scheme these represent various stages along the way. He will thus describe them, remaining within the basic framework, as lying between 'psora and sycosis' or 'sycosis and syphilis', with variations of these as appropriate. Similarly with the cancer and tubercular miasms, these are merely reflections of the three fundamental miasms acting together in a fixed and consistent way that produces an identifiable disease pattern.

The idea of an infectious connection to the miasms still persists to some degree, and there are, as a consequence, ideas about such as distemper or rabies miasms arising as a result of vaccination or exposure to infection.

The whole range of responses to disease is expressed by some people in terms of the miasms, and comparisons are made with the changing physiological processes and balances that occur throughout life. This can initially make the subject very confusing, but it must be realised that all these interpretations are only attempts to explain and expand the Hahnemannian concept of chronic disease in the light of modern knowledge and thought.

A Model for the Miasms

The areas of broad physiological function that are at the root of both Grauvogl's and Hahnemann's classification can be divided into three types. Firstly, there is the need for an overall control and orchestration of all functions, and the maintenance of a proper internal environment. Secondly, the creation of new cells and tissues to replace worn out or damaged parts, and to meet special requirements at particular times, such as reproduction. Finally, there is the need for the removal of damaged tissues, toxic materials and the destruction of foreign invaders. The body is continuously operating in all of these three ways on both a pathological and functional level. The interplay of the functions is essential for life and the balance between them is constantly changing to meet the needs of the moment, but a fluctuating equilibrium between them is always present in health.

This implies that no one function must become too predominant for too long, although there will be times when it is necessary for one of them to be more active than the others – for example, the elevation of the body temperature and the increase in phagacytosis that is triggered during the immune response to infection. However, if that response does not settle down once it is no longer needed, or the body becomes conditioned to a particular exaggerated or inappropriate response at all times, then the essential balance is lost. What is then seen is the body functioning in an unbalanced way, which manifests as what is recognised homeopathically as a miasm.

Thus one way of viewing the miasms is to regard them as basic physiological functions of the body that have become distorted. The manifestation of a miasm can be regarded as an indication of a lack of balance in the equilibrium that is essential for health, and for as long as such an imbalance persists the body will be incapable of reacting normally to any challenge.

Each of the miasms corresponds to one of the basic functions of the body that has become exaggerated. Pathologically the main characteristics of the three miasms are now thought of as:

Psora	Deficiency, atrophy, failure of function
Sycosis	Excess
Syphilis	Destruction, perversion.

An exaggeration of the control and homeostatic function in the body becomes psora; that of new tissue production causes excess, which manifests as sycosis, while the body's overenthusiastic removal of debris becomes the destructive force that is recognised as syphilis.

In a perfectly healthy individual (if such exists), the physiological forces are in balance and remain so. It is, however, a fluctuating balance, constantly changing to meet the needs of the moment. All challenges and bodily requirements will be met by temporary increases in those physiological activities that are necessary to restore the equilibrium, and they will function to the degree and in the order required by the situation. Once the challenge has been successfully dealt with, the physiology returns to its previous state of balance. This is what happens during routine homeostasis and acute infections.

However, in chronic disease the balance of the physiological forces has become unbalanced, and one will have become predominant in relation to the others. The required response to any situation will therefore be unbalanced. The other two activities do not cease to operate, but their action is masked and distorted by the dominant partner. The term 'dis-ease' represents this imbalance. In these circumstances the body is incapable of reacting normally, but will respond to all circumstances in a way that predominantly reflects the now major influence. Miasms can therefore be viewed as functional disturbances of normal physiology that have attained pathological proportions due to imbalances within the system.

Creation and Inheritance of Miasms

Suppression of the natural disease process, as discussed in Chapters 4 and 5, is at the heart of the creation of miasms. Within the model, the restoration of the normal balance of the physiological forces after illness is dependent on the working through of Hering's Law, and for as long as this is allowed to continue no major inequalities between the physiological forces will be created. However, if the normal direction of Hering's law is blocked by inappropriate treatment, then the process of cure is turned in on itself and, if the block continues or is repeated, will reverse and take the disease into deeper levels. The blocking will result in a cessation of the curative process and the creation of an abnormal balance between the basic physiological influences. Because of the reversal of the healing process, this abnormal balance will become the new basis from which future adjustments to challenge are made, and because it is itself abnormal, all adjustments arising from it will also be abnormal. Thus a clinical miasm can be established.

The second way in which a miasm may be produced is when the system is subjected to too severe a challenge for it to cope with at an early stage of its development. The immaturity of such a system means that it will not have established the necessary long-term balance between its functions. Indeed, in the young animal there will be the increased activity of cell creation necessary to ensure growth. A severe shock to the system at this stage may result in a permanent imbalance between the physiological forces, thus creating a miasm. This will influence the reaction of the body to the further challenges that will inevitably occur in the course of normal life.

Finally, if the system is continuously exposed to the same challenge, it will be necessary for it to respond to the challenge in the same way every time. Thus the system can become conditioned to respond to all challenges in the same way, irrespective of whether it is an appropriate response or not.

What are often referred to as the 'new' miasms – that is, the more recently recognised clinical entities of which the cancer and tubercular miasms are the most accepted – may be regarded as situations in which the imbalance of function in an individual system has become a fixed functional entity rather than the three separate but inter-connected forces of control, new growth and removal. The exact nature of the imbalance will be different for each new miasm, but it will always be constant for that miasm.

Why this imbalance has become established will depend on several factors. One is the overwhelming and continuous exposure, usually over several generations, of a population to a particular infection (e.g. tuberculosis). Another is the continuous suppressive treatment of disease. Cancer as a disease is characterised by the proliferation of abnormal tissues and invasion and destruction of healthy tissue. The miasmatic influences involved in these processes are sycosis and syphilis, and hence cancer is regarded miasmatically as being predominantly syphilitic with a significant sycotic element. Clinically, tuberculosis shows wasting, weakness and a failure to overcome the infection and thrive. Miasmatically, wasting is syphilitic, whilst weakness and failure are psoric, and thus the miasm is considered to be a mixture of psora and syphilis.

Clinical experience shows that both the individual basic influences and these new fixed entities can be passed from generation to generation. In many cases eczema is known to affect different members of the same family, and it is well recognised that there are 'cancer families' in which the disease in some form occurs regularly without any common precipitating cause. Indeed, the reinforcing of a pattern inherited from a previous generation results, as might be expected, in a stronger pattern. However, although miasmatic tendencies can be seen in conventionally defined inherited conditions, miasmatic influences also appear to be capable of passing through the generations by some mechanism other that conventional genetics. It has been suggested that modifications in the component make-up of the DNA result from the creation of a miasmatic influence in the individual, and that this is then passed on (Elliott). Another idea is that the DNA can function as an electro-magnetic receiver/transmitter and what are being passed down the generations are energy imprints (Subramanian). This has obvious similarities with some of the ideas concerning the creation of high potency remedies, and emphasises the fact that in homeopathy we are dealing with energy and function rather than material and pathology.

Recognising Miasms

In order for miasms to be used as clinical tools it is necessary for the pattern of a particular miasm's activity to be recognised. It must always be remembered that in every case there will be symptoms that do not fit into the pattern because they are due to the activity of the other forces. It is also possible to have two active miasms in a case at the same time. Nevertheless, there will be one that is predominant and this is the pattern that will be imposed on the whole symptom picture.

As with other prescribing strategies, it is always necessary to take account of the presenting symptom picture when selecting a remedy. During the course of (successful) treatment, the pattern may change as one dominant miasm is dealt with and another takes its place. This is then prescribed for based on the new presenting picture. However, the fact of there being a strong miasmatic pattern is part of the symptom picture, and the correct remedy will correspond to the presenting miasmatic pattern (see below).

The following broad indications will guide the prescriber towards a particular miasm.

Psora

Due to the failure and the weakness that are in the picture, psoric conditions are those that are described as 'hypo'. Atrophy, weakness and lack of production are seen. Failure to recover following illness is a feature, with slow healing of wounds. There is restlessness and sensitivity, based in large part on fears and anxieties. Conditions tend to be < before noon and > afternoon, although this time feature is not so well marked as the time connections of the other two miasms. Conditions are improved by physiological discharges such as the passage of water or faeces. This also includes perspiration in those species where that is seen, although because of the poor control of the system this tends to occur on only slight exertion and in some cases even at rest in moderate temperatures. There is a general sensitivity to cold and conditions are < for it. The general lack of reactivity results in a tendency towards pain*less* conditions, especially in connection with the bowels, and the animal may be unaffected by constipation with no attempt to pass the motion. The appetite may be poor or ravenous but the digestion is weak, with much resulting flatulence. The skin will show irritation, which can be intense, but without any pathology; the coat will be dry (hyposecretion) and the only lesions seen will be as a result of self-mutilation.

Paradoxically there may be fever, but this will usually be out of proportion in some way to the severity of the challenge, and represents either an aspect of the lack of control or a failure of function. Similarly, allergy is considered to have a major psoric component and this is also a reflection of the inability to control a sycotic response.

Discharges are thin and watery with an offensive odour, and general odours from the body, when present, are also offensive.

The suppression of a psoric response will drive the disease process primarily into the nervous system. In its pure psoric form this will show as paralysis, but linked to sycosis may appear as epilepsy.

Sycosis

'Hyper' is the type of reaction that is seen in sycosis. Excessive growth of tissues and overproduction of secretions on the physical level, and extreme reactions in the mental sphere, are characteristic. Although the manifestation of sycotic disease generally has an extreme element in the symptomology, conditions are often slow in onset. There is generally a strong connection with water, showing either as upsets to the fluid balance of the body, or a general symptom and modality of < damp. A combination of this and the extreme mental reactions that are seen means that animals are often very upset by storms. There is irritation of any of the mucous surfaces, which become congested and in-flamed with a resultant increase in the discharges from them. The discharges are thick, yellow/green in colour and will stain any material with which they come in contact. Any smell associated with them is often fishy. Perspiration when it occurs also tends to have a strong, often sweet smell, and is copious. Conditions are > pathological dis-charges, as in a case of pyometra that brightens generally once it becomes open.

Skin conditions may be either irritant or non-irritant and are charac-terised by thickening and increased pigmentation. Warts and benign lumps are seen, whilst cysts represent both the thickening and increase of tissues and the retention of fluid. Many infections of the ears are predominantly sycotic, especially if accompanied by a fishy-smelling discharge. Claws, nails and hooves are often affected and are usually thickened; sometimes the growth of them is so rapid that the quality suffers and softness and cracking is seen.

The miasm is marked by pain*ful* abdominal conditions. Colic and spasm of the internal organs are part of the picture, and any associated diarrhoea is likely to have an explosive quality to it coupled with a degree of urgency. Inflammation is sycotic and when joints are involved there is often the formation of exostoses. There is a tendency to the formation of calculi in the gall bladder, kidneys and bladder.

Both the general symptom and the local modality of < from sunrise to sunset is a distinct feature, being more marked than the corresponding aspect of the psoric miasm.

There is a marked affinity with both the urinary and genital systems, and sycotic conditions in the body will often find an outlet via these. Suppression of the miasm tends to drive it primarily into these two systems.

The characteristic pattern of disease is often shown in birds, who have a strong sycotic element in their make-up. Disease conditions tend to be hidden for as long as possible and then to progress rapidly to an extreme form.

Syphilis

This is Nature's 'self-destruct button'. Conditions are described as 'dys', with deviation of function and tissues. Ulceration, haemorrhage, destruction and perversion of both function and tissues are seen. An improvement in the general condition of the patient is often seen when ulceration appears on the skin. Chronic infections are seen with pus and blood, and wounds fail to heal because of underlying infection, while there is swelling and ulceration of glandular tissues. Mentally there is a tendency to be morbid and dull with much depression produced by illness, especially due to pain. A definite time connection of < from sunset to sunrise exists. Extremes of temperature will upset patients but conditions are generally > cold. A preference for cold food and drink is not perhaps a major observation in animals but it can occasionally be identified, especially when it shows as a craving for things such as ice cream or a desire to drink water straight from the tap before it is warmed by the ambient temperature. Physiological discharges result in aggravation of syphilitic conditions.

Many syphilitic states are pain*ful*, and this may be intense; but at the other end of the scale they may become pain*less* due to destruction of tissues, this being seen mainly in the skin. Discolourations of the skin other than pigmentation are syphilitic and are usually red/brown and roughly circular in shape.

The organs of sense are susceptible to the miasm. Infectious conditions of both the middle and external ear are seen and many eye conditions have a strong syphilitic element; most are marked by photophobia.

Congenital abnormalities that are characterised by deformities of limbs or organs are usually syphilitic. (Complete failure of development, in contrast, is psoric.) The skeleton is particularly affected, with the hips especially so.

Destruction is not confined to diseased tissues, and the destruction of healthy tissues is also seen. Thus in syphilitic conditions there is often weight loss (which may be severe), which cannot be accounted for by failures of diet or appetite. Dental neck lesions are syphilitic, as they involve invasive decay and destruction of the tissues of the tooth.

Suppression of the external manifestations of the miasm will drive it into the brain, the meninges and the bones.

Anti-Miasmatic Remedies

Linked to the concept of miasmatic disease is the concept of anti-miasmatic remedies. These are remedies that have a major part of their remedy picture closely reflecting that of one particular miasm. Accordingly, each is especially useful in treating conditions in which the appropriate miasm predominates. However, in all disease situations all three miasms are still acting to some degree, and this is mirrored by the presence of symptoms of all three influences in every remedy. The proportion of symptoms will, of course, vary with individual remedies. Thus what are regarded as strongly anti-miasmatic remedies should always be thought of as only being *predominantly* rather than completely so. Another confusion that can arise is that homeopaths almost invariably qualify these remedies solely by the adjective of the miasm; for example, Thuja is usually described as being a 'sycotic remedy'. Although this is the accepted convention, it must never be forgotten that the true description should be 'a predominantly anti-sycotic remedy'.

Examples of other major remedies that are generally considered, from clinical experience, to be linked to particular miasms are Calcarea Carbonica and Lycopodium for psora and Aurum Metallicum and Phytolacca for syphilis. Phosphorus is linked with the tubercular miasm, while Sepia and Causticum are other remedies reflecting the sycotic miasm. Sulphur is often mainly linked to the psoric miasm but many consider it to be more of a tri-miasmatic remedy, that is, one reflecting the miasms in roughly equal proportions. The above is by no means an exhaustive list, and it must be remembered that even these remedies will show definite symptoms associated with the other miasms.

In addition to this type of remedy there are the miasmatic nosodes. (The whole concept of nosodes is discussed in Chapter 12.) These are the most closely linked of any remedies to their particular miasms. Their source material is closely associated with the appropriate disease process, but equally important is the fact that they contain an element of the response to the disease process. Whilst they very much reflect the essence of the miasms they are also remedies in their own right and can on occasion be used as such. Their main area of use, however, is in the treatment of chronic disease associated with a particular miasm, and they are often used as inter-current remedies as a means of overcoming the obstacle to cure that the miasm can represent.

References

Banerjea, S.K. (2003) *Miasmatic Diagnosis*. New Delhi: B. Jain Publishers.

Chambers Twentieth Century Dictionary. Edinburgh: Chambers.

Elliott, M. (1996) Possible inheritance of miasms. *BAHVS Newsletter*, Spring.

Hallamaa, R.E. et al. (2001) Treatment of equine summer eczema with an autogenous serum preparation, possibly effected by inductional lipid signals. *Deutsche Zeitschrift für Onkologie* **33**, 57-62.

Ortega, P.S. (1980) *Notes on the Miasms*. New Delhi: National Homeopathic Pharmacy.

Saxton, J.G.G. (in preparation) *Miasms as Practical Tools*. Beaconsfield: Beaconsfield Publishers.

Sonnenschmidt, R. (2001) Lecture on avian homeopathy. *Presented at the BAHVS conference*, Harper Adams College, Newport, Shropshire, UK.

Spink, F. (2001) Miasms and toxins. In: Reyner, J.H. (ed) *Psionic Medicine*, pp. 94-106. Saffron Walden: C.W. Daniel.

Subramanian, R. (2001) *Miasms. Their Effect on the Human Organism*. New Delhi: B. Jain Publishers.

Chapter 12

Isopathy and the Use of Nosodes

The term *isopathy* is used to describe the employment of potentised remedies prepared from substances responsible for the disease being treated. The word is derived from the Greek *'iso'* meaning 'equal'. It is a matter for discussion as to whether isopathy should be addressed in a textbook of homeopathy, as strictly speaking its definition excludes it from consideration within that sphere of medicine. However, as it has been developed by homeopaths and its acceptance has grown alongside the development of homeopathy, isopathy is generally considered to be a part of the armoury of the homeopath.

A *nosode* is a potentised remedy prepared from diseased tissue or the product of disease (from the Greek *nosos* = disease, *eidos* = like). (Strictly speaking, a remedy is only homeopathic when prescribed for a patient whose symptomatology corresponds to that of the remedy – until then it is simply a 'potentised' remedy.)

Hahnemann himself prepared remedies from diseased tissue, foremost of which were the so-called 'miasmatic' nosodes, Psorinum, Medorrhinum and Syphilinum. Since then many others have been prepared, not only from human or animal derivatives but also occasionally from plant sources. Examples of the latter include Secale (prepared from rye affected by ergot fungus) and Ustilago (corn smut). In addition, with the advent of microbiological culturing techniques, remedies have been prepared from pure cultures of infectious agents. It should be noted that the latter do not contain any of the host tissue and may therefore differ from their host-derived counterparts. In order to distinguish them from other nosodes, remedies derived from pure cultures are sometimes erroneously referred to as *homeopathic vaccines* or, more correctly, *pathodes*.

The major nosodes have undergone thorough provings and their use in veterinary homeopathy on this basis is no different from that of any other homeopathic remedy. However, somewhere between 1831 and 1833 Joseph Lux, a German veterinary surgeon, investigated the idea of using nosodes in the treatment of the specific disease from which they were derived. Lux used Anthracinum in the treatment of cattle affected by anthrax and he is credited with coining the term *isopathy* to describe this field of therapy.

Nosodes are further classified on the basis of the source and recipient. An *isonosode* is a potentised remedy made from diseased tissues or products of disease from the same group of patients/animals. An *autonosode* is a potentised remedy made from diseased tissues or products of disease from the same patient.

Bearing in mind the above definition of isopathy, the use of 'disease-producing agents' other than those of an infectious nature may be included in the concept. Allergens, for instance, may be potentised and used in desensitising programmes. These are sometimes, rather clumsily, termed *allergodes*. Stretching the definition slightly, there is a whole range of medicines available which are derived from the potentisation of organs and tissues from healthy individuals (usually human). These medicines are termed *sarcodes*, defined as 'homeopathic remedies made from healthy glandular or tissue extracts', and are used in organ support regimes, usually in conjunction with other levels of homeopathic prescribing. Their use was first advocated by Hering in 1834.

Finally, under the heading of isopathy comes the term *tautopathy*, 'a form of isotherapy, using homeopathic remedies prepared from allopathic medicine, in order to counteract the side effects caused by that particular medication'.

USES OF ISOPATHY

'Never Well Since' (NWS)

A clear causality in the history of a patient presented for homeopathy is 'like gold-dust', such are its implications for success, and this is no less true if the instigating factor of the disease has been on the physical, rather than the mental plane. If an infectious disease can be identified as the cause of subsequent illness, then the use of a nosode of that disease can not only be helpful but occasionally also essential in the successful homeopathic treatment of that patient. The infection may of course have been deliberately introduced in the form of a vaccine; if available, a homeopathic remedy derived from the vaccine itself may be used in this situation. This latter could well be regarded as tautopathy, and if the exciting cause is identified as a particular allopathic medicine, then the use of a homeopathic preparation derived from that medicine will be beneficial. This is particularly effective if the animal is suffering from recognised side effects of the medicine.

Desensitisation

Where a specific allergen is implicated, either from laboratory investigations or circumstantial evidence, this may be potentised and used in a desensitising programme.

Treatment of Active Disease

Where a specific disease is present in an individual, the use of the nosode from that disease may be employed. However, if the disease is unidentified, isopathy can still be employed by preparing an autonosode from pathological emanations such as nasal discharges or diarrhoea. Non-specific infectious disease may be countered by the use of autonosodes prepared from blood and/or urine; this latter technique, though rarely practised by the authors, is considered by its advocates to confer a general improvement in immune response, whatever the cause of the infectious disease. However, a word of caution may be appropriate here – it is the authors' experience that treatment of active disease with the specific nosode can result in a significant aggravation of the symptoms more frequently than would be expected from a purely homeopathic approach.

Prophylaxis

It is generally accepted among homeopaths, medical and veterinary, that when the nosode of a specific infectious disease is administered to a healthy individual a protective effect ensues. Anecdotal evidence and veterinary homeopaths' experience, including that of the authors, seems to confirm that present dosage regimes of homeopathic nosodes in this way have some protective effect. However, there is as yet no evidence in the form of custom-designed trials to support this and the area remains contentious. Further discussion will be found in Chapter 14.

Epidemic/epizootic disease

Opportunities for using nosodes in this situation are rare in veterinary medicine; the advent of canine parvovirus in the 1970s and the 2001 Foot and Mouth disease (FMD) epizootic are exceptions, although in neither case are there any records of the use of homeopathic nosodes for prophylaxis. Indeed, the use of nosodes for the prophylaxis of a notifiable disease such as FMD would be unethical, although it might be considered in countries where the disease is endemic.

The pattern of Foot and Mouth disease is, of course, influenced by the disease control policies of national governments. The slaughter approach to control, with or without temporary vaccination, aims at a disease-free national herd. This means that when outbreaks occur they follow an epizootic pattern. In parts of the world where such policies are not followed, the disease is often of a more enzootic nature.

Endemic/enzootic disease

This represents the most common form of prophylaxis employing nosodes. Combined nosodes of all the common infectious diseases are available from the major homeopathic pharmacies. Ideally these will have been produced from disease material, though there is sometimes uncertainty as to whether pure strains of the organism have been used as source material.

One of the advantages of the prophylactic use of nosodes is that they can be prepared for any disease as long as there is disease material to present to a homeopathic pharmacy. Consequently, nosodes have long been prepared from such diseases as Feline Infectious Peritonitis and Feline Immunodeficiency Virus where no conventional vaccine has been available.

Once again, in small animals, there is little evidence to support the use of nosodes in this way but one of us (Saxton 1991) has documented significant effect in reducing the incidence of distemper in a welfare kennels by the use of distemper nosode.

In the case of farm animals several trials have been performed, notably in the control of mastitis in dairy cows (Day 1986).

In face of an outbreak (pre-emptive)

This is another area where there is documented evidence of efficacy of use of nosodes. An outbreak of kennel cough in a boarding kennels was managed by the administration of a nosode; incidence of disease was markedly reduced (Day 1987). Isopathy therefore represents an extremely useful tool in these circumstances. A generic nosode may be available immediately from a homeopathic pharmacist; alternatively one may be prepared within a very short time from material collected from affected animals – indeed, it is not even necessary to have a specific diagnosis for therapy or prophylaxis to begin.

Organotherapy

Where the pathology of the specific organ is known, administration of a sarcode can have a beneficial effect on the organ; generally a low potency preparation is given over a long period of time. Interestingly, and of significance in therapy, is the observation that a potency-specific effect exists: potencies above 7c appear to reduce the activity of an organ while those of under 7c are considered to stimulate it. (The effects of using exactly 7c are uncertain.) Thyroidinum (a sarcode prepared from bovine thyroid gland) might therefore be administered at 6c for hypothyroid states, and at 30c for hyperthyroidism. Further discussion of this phenomenon is to be found on pages 93 and 256.

Bowel Nosodes

These are specialised nosodes prepared from specific organisms cultured from human gut contents; a full discussion of their development and usage is contained in the following chapter.

Prescription on Miasmatic Criteria

Where a clear miasmatic pattern runs through a case, and especially if it is uncertain which homeopathic medicine represents the simillimum for the patient, the technique of administering the appropriate miasmatic nosode can be of value. If the miasmatic diagnosis is accurate, this will invariably have some beneficial effect. In addition, when the patient is reassessed some time after the administration of the miasmatic nosode, it is usual for their symptomatology to have changed. This then allows a more accurate prescription to be made on strictly homeopathic principles. The benficial effect of miasmatic nosodes prescribed on such criteria can often be marked, although another remedy, selected on more classical criteria, will almost always be needed to complete the cure. The corollary to this is that if a patient has not responded to one or more seemingly well indicated remedies, a miasmatic nosode may be of help. Not surprisingly, therefore, the phrase 'when well indicated remedies fail to act' is often found within the descriptions of these nosodes in the materia medica.

The Miasmatic Nosodes

Psorinum

Manufactured by potentising the contents of a human scabies vesicle, Psorinum represents the psoric miasm. As such there is itchiness, deficiency and gloom. The Psorinum patient is anxious and melancholy, itchy, smelly and chilly. Indeed the chilliness is extreme, the dog or cat hugging the fire in winter and stretching out in the hot sun in summer. Psorinum also loves to be covered and will burrow under bedding to keep warm. (Compare and contrast this with the other archetype of psora, Sulphur, which generally shows aversion to heat.) Appetite is often ravenous, especially at night, but the patient rarely puts on weight. Not surprisingly, considering the source material, symptoms centre around the skin. There is alopecia, and the Psorinum dog has greasy, itchy skin; indeed, in the repertory there is a small rubric 'despair from itching' in which Psorinum is the only medicine in bold type. However, bathing may actually ameliorate the symptoms and the dog requiring Psorinum will often attempt to clean itself by constantly licking itself, the feet in particular. These attempts are, however, unsuccessful and Psorinum retains its filthy demeanour despite all endeavours by patient or owner to the contrary. All discharges are offensive, be they the result of otitis, diarrhoea or urogenital disease.

Keynotes: Chilly, itchy and smelly.

Medorrhinum

Prepared from human gonorrhoea, Medorrhinum represents the sycotic miasm. The overactivity of this miasm is reflected in profuse discharges from any orifice, excrescences on the skin and a predilection for joints and urogenital system. Mentally the patient is hurried and may be aggressive. Medorrhinum tends to be on the chilly side, but more marked than this is the sensitivity to damp conditions; all symptoms are worse in damp weather. In addition there is the rather unusual amelioration by the seaside. This rubric ('Generals; air; seaside; air at the; ameliorates') is shared by other medicines, amongst them Tuberculinum and Carcinosin, but nowhere is it more marked than in Medorrhinum. Joint symptoms include swelling of joints and exostoses, and pain is ameliorated by motion. Urogenital symptoms include pyometra, vaginitis, cystitis, balanoposthitis and prostatic disease. The skin is prone to warts and other benign tumours, especially in the genital and perineal areas. Symptoms tend to be worse during the daytime.

Keynotes: Profuse discharges, urogenital and arthritic symptoms.

Syphilinum

Representing the syphilitic miasm, Syphilinum (sometimes referred to as 'Lueticum' or 'Luesinum') stands for destruction. Mentally there is hopeless despair and fear of disease. There is also an issue around death; this may be fear of death, or, more easily observed in animals, a desire to kill. Whereas Medorrhinum will show aggression almost as a way of shedding excess energy, Syphilinum will look like it would kill – and indeed sometimes will succeed in killing – another animal. Destructive processes on the local level are centred around bone and allied structures. In humans there is tooth decay below the gum margins and this may also be observed in dogs; in cats the counterpart is the erosive odontoclastic lesion. Destruction of bone in the nasal cavities leads to chronic nasal discharges and nasal and oral cancer. Eyes are also affected, with ulceration, keratitis and iridocyclitis. Mucous membranes are ulcerated and ulcers may appear on the skin; also recurrent abscesses. Symptoms are worse between sunset and sunrise.

Keynotes: Ulceration, destruction of bone, chronic eye symptoms.

Tuberculinum Bovinum

There are several homeopathic preparations representing the tubercular miasm, however Tuberculinum Bovinum (Tub. Bov.), prepared from tuberculous bovine lung, is the most commonly used. The theme of Tuberculinum is changeability. Symptoms are constantly changing and there is an innate desire in the patient for change; the cat or dog gets bored with the same food and will only eat properly when the flavour or brand is periodically changed; symptoms of skin disease come and go within minutes; joint pains wander from limb to limb. Not surprisingly, Tuberculinum centres on the lungs, being associated with chronic respiratory disease of many forms. Upper respiratory disease also occurs, with chronic nasal discharge. Mentally the need for per-petual change is reflected in the restlessness which Tuberculinum exhibits. Never still at home and constantly wandering round the con-sulting room, the Tuberculinum dog will escape to roam the streets if given half the chance.

Add to this the destructiveness (on both the emotional and pathological planes) which this medicine contains, and we have the typical picture of a lean, hyperactive dog who destroys the home when left alone, and escapes at the first opportunity; the word which sums this up is 'delinquency'. Chronic or recurrent tonsillitis with swelling of the lymph glands, indeed lymphadenopathy in any site, and chronic diarrhoea, especially in young animals, are some of the more common local symptoms. There is usually also an issue around milk; either an abnormal craving, an aversion, or intolerance.

Better for the open air and worse for getting wet, especially getting the feet wet, thus the Tuberculinum dog won't walk through puddles.

Keynotes: Thin despite ravenous appetite, rapid changeability of symptoms, chronic respiratory disease, 'delinquency'.

Carcinosin

There are several nosodes prepared from human carcinomata, the most commonly used being Carcinosin (from breast cancer) and Scirrhinum (from liver cancer). Carcinosin is generally taken as being most representative of the cancer archetype, although cancer is perhaps the most difficult of the miasmatic patterns to identify, there being so much suppression in its picture. There is some element of control or being controlled in Carcinosin, so it is often indicated in dogs which have been over-trained; in fact they are so 'well-trained' that they don't dare put a foot wrong. Highly sensitive, they are obedient and submissive. The Carcinosin patient is fastidious and may have an almost unique love of thunderstorms; Carcinosin dogs will actually enjoy looking out of a window to watch a storm, and only Sepia shares the rubric 'Loves thunderstorms'. Carcinosin generally dislikes heat and may prefer open air so may be confused with Pulsatilla, being also mild and yielding. However, the affectionate nature of Pulsatilla is less marked in Carcinosin and in fact Carcinosin may be intolerant of consolation.

Carcinosin is a relative newcomer to veterinary prescribing and it is only in recent years that it has been studied in any depth. Local symptoms which have responded to it vary from mental and emotional problems to chronic skin disease, but its major use remains as an intercurrent remedy in the treatment of cancer; indeed, one of the main pointers to the use of Carcinosin is the presence of cancer in the patient's own or family history. In this context, breeders often seem to know about cancer in the line, despite the fact that they may be reluctant to exchange information about other conditions.

Keynotes: Timidity, fastidiousness, love of thunderstorms, history of cancer, control.

References

Day, C.E.I. (1986) Clinical trials in bovine mastitis using nosodes for prevention. *International Journal of Veterinary Homeopathy* **1**, 15.

Day, C.E.I. (1987) Isopathic prevention of kennel cough. *International Journal of Veterinary Homeopathy* **2**, 57.

Saxton, J. (1991) Use of distemper nosode in disease control. *International Journal of Veterinary Homeopathy* **15**, 8.

Swayne, J. (ed.) (2000) *International Dictionary of Homeopathy*. Edinburgh: Churchill Livingstone.

Yasgur, J. (1998) *Homeopathic Dictionary and Holistic Health Reference* (4th edn). Greenville, PA: Van Hoy Publishers.

Chapter 13

The Bowel Nosodes

Development of the Bowel Nosodes

The bowel nosodes are a group of eleven homeopathic remedies that have as their source material certain bacteria which occur in the bowels in particular circumstances linked to the healing process.

Although they are a purely homeopathic concept, their origins lie in the work of conventional immunologists during the early years of the twentieth century. The best known of these was Dr Edward Bach, who later devoted himself to the development of the Flower Remedies. The other major workers in the field were Drs John and Elizabeth Paterson, who were active at the same time and largely took over the project. Others were involved at times, and made valuable contributions, but then moved on. The nomenclature of the bowel nosodes can be confusing, but the inclusion of the names 'Bach' and 'Paterson' in the terminology found in some texts indicates the worker who first developed the particular nosode. The term 'Co.' when encountered in remedy names stands for 'compound', as each remedy is based on a combination of different bacterial strains.

The nosodes are derived in the main from gram-negative, non-lactose fermenting bacilli that are found in the bowels of patients exhibiting certain clinical patterns. The use of lactose as a means of classification is primarily a laboratory technique, but it should be noted that lactose is the only sugar of animal origin that is used routinely in the laboratory, and a link has been established between lactose and the action in the bowels of *Bacillus acidophilus* (Yale 1921). In view of the current ideas on, and usage of, probiotics, this link offers a possible explanation of the mechanisms involved in the bowel nosode story. It is certainly true that chronic disease processes produce changes in the alimentary mucosa that allow changes in the composition of the bowel flora.

The original conventional immunological work was concerned with the use of autogenous vaccines. Chronic disease was viewed as essentially an intestinal toxaemia, the toxins being produced by the non-lactose fermenting bacteria that were being found in the bowels, with a

147

basic fault in the permeability of the intestinal mucosa allowing them to be absorbed. For many years, after his introduction to homeopathy, Dr Bach regarded psora as being essentially intestinal toxaemia. The presence of these bacilli in the bowels was attributed to dietary factors and although an increase in the proportion of raw food in the diet was recommended, the main thrust of treatment was via a vaccination regime. During the course of this work Dr Bach moved to the London Homeopathic Hospital (1919) as its bacteriologist, and was thus exposed to the homeopathic way of thought. He and Dr Wheeler applied this to the vaccination routine, employing a homeopathic concept of dosage to the treatments. Observations from the monitoring of the necessary faecal samples was the start of the bowel nosodes, but the initial thinking was still governed by the 'cause and effect' thinking associated with the 'germ theory' approach to disease.

A crucial fact had been established by 1924 by Dr Wheeler. This was that faecal counts from clinical cases often showed only low or non-existent levels of non-lactose fermenting bacilli. Repeated samples taken during the course of an illness showed both positive and negative phases of production of the bacilli, and these phases were consistently related to the state of health of the patient. Successful treatment resulted in a marked increase in the numbers of non-lactose fermenting bacilli present, which then reduced again and finally disappeared. Even without treatment it was found that there were both positive and negative phases to the production of the non-lactose fermenters, which matched the varying condition of the patient. A high level of the relevant bacteria would coincide with an improvement in the patient's condition, while the numbers reduced again when there was a relapse. It was subsequently shown that when successful treatment was given, the increase in the numbers of non-lactose fermenters in the bowel flora followed this same pattern, and the change usually occurred within 10–14 days of a beneficial treatment (cf. vaccination), and was often maintained for a considerable period of time. Cases were recorded of non-lactose fermenters persisting in excess of a year. However, in cases where a cure was achieved, the non-lactose fermenters would finally disappear while health would be maintained. In contrast, other associated work showed that the effect of diet on the intestinal flora could take a considerable time to appear, and was only maintained for as long as the diet was persevered with. As a result of these and other observations, by 1928 Dr Bach was wondering:

'Whether these organisms (the NLFB) are the cause of, the result of, or an attempt by the body to cure, disease?'

Dr Bach was never able to fully free himself from the idea that the non-lactose fermenters were in some way pathogenic, partly perhaps because his mind was already turning towards plants as the primary therapeutic agents. It was at this point that he left the work and moved on into his development of the Flower Remedies. The Drs Paterson in Glasgow, who had been working on the same lines now became the focus. Although Dr Bach had a great sympathy for homeopathy he was never a practising homeopath, and his treatments had not been solely based on remedies. The Patersons were homeopaths and approached the whole subject from an entirely homeopathic point of view. One of their concerns was the limitations of classical germ theory and the role of host susceptibility in disease. They also had the Hahnemannian concept of chronic disease as a deep-seated, multi-symptom entity.

By giving consideration to these concerns they were able to clarify the question of the exact nature of the phenomenon which was being observed. They came to the conclusion that 'the non-lactose fermenting organisms found in the bowels are the <u>result</u> of a vital reaction on the part of the body tissues.'

The above underlining has been made to emphasise the crucial part this conclusion plays in the understanding of the whole subject. It should also be noted that in the above quotation the term vital is used in the homeopathic sense – that is, involving the vital force. We have seen elsewhere that the influence of the vital force always acts so as to restore the balance that we call health. Hence anything that results from this must be part of the curative reaction of the body.

That the production of the non-lactose fermenting bacilli in the bowels is a result of the body's response to disease is shown by two facts. Firstly that the production of the bacilli is increased by the administration of a treatment having a beneficial effect on the presenting picture, and secondly that this is accompanied by an improvement in the general health of the patient.

One of the earliest observations in relation to the bowel nosodes was the establishment of the pattern of positive and negative phases. In chronic disease there is a constantly fluctuating balance between the action of the vital force (curative) and the disease process. The variations in the levels of the relevant bacilli can be considered as indicative of this fluctuation.

The establishment of this relationship has of course resolved the dilemma of pathogenicity that so concerned Dr Bach, and indeed others, in the early days. One of the reasons that Dr Bach left the work and began his investigations into the Flower Remedies was that he was looking for an approach to curing disease that had no possible hint of pathogenicity about it. It is important to be clear on this point, as in modern terminology we are discussing gram-negative members of the Enterobacteriacae family, including certain salmonella species. But there is no pathological risk in this direction as the bacteria involved are essentially saprophytic in conventional terms. It must also be borne in mind that the bowel nosodes are not, in the strict sense of the term, nosodes at all. Although they are produced from bacteria associated with disease, the presence of the bacteria is part of the *curative* action of the body, and is not associated with the pathogenic action of any causative or trigger agent.

The eleven bowel nosodes are the remedies Morgan Pure, Morgan Gaertner (these two often combined as Morgan Bach), Proteus, Dysentery Co., Gaertner Bach, Sycotic Co., Faecalis, Mutabile, Bacillus No. 7, Bacillus No. 10 and Coccal Co. Further details are given later in this chapter.

The Associated Remedies

The relationship between the normal homeopathic remedies and the bowel nosodes is not quite the same as the remedy relationships that are spoken of in other contexts. That is why the term 'associated remedies' is preferable, although they are sometimes called 'related' or 'indicated' remedies. The appearance of non-lactose fermenting bacilli in the bacterial flora of the bowels only follows the application of a beneficial treatment. In homeopathic terms this means a correctly chosen remedy. But it was found that the particular types of non-lactose fermenting bacilli which appeared could be linked to treatment with specific remedies, and that successful treatment with those remedies always resulted in the same bacilli emerging.

This connection between the administration of a well-chosen and effective remedy and the appearance of specific non-lactose fermenting bacilli has another aspect. The selection of the remedy is based on the presenting symptom picture of the patient. There is therefore a definite homeopathic relationship between the symptom picture and the appropriate bacilli that appear in the bowels. This means that there is in fact a three-way interactive relationship that can be expressed visually as:

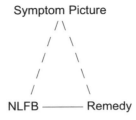

Because of this interaction, the possibility of using the bacilli as homeopathic remedies arises. Dr John Paterson expressed it as:

> 'If Natrum Mur. causes *B. proteus* (a NLFB) to appear in the stool, may not the remedy be efficacious in the patient yielding *B. proteus* in high percentage?' (as a result of treatment)

The above triangle therefore becomes:

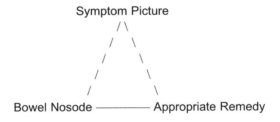

It is this interrelationship that forms the basis for the concept of the related remedies. From this relationship it is also clear that the bowel nosodes are truly homeopathic.

The list at the end of the chapter shows the links that have been established between some of the remedies and the eleven bowel nosodes (the terms related, associated, or indicated remedies are often interchanged). The nomenclature remains the same as was originally devised. In practice, as already mentioned, Morgan Pure and Morgan Gaertner are often mixed together to form a remedy known as Morgan Bach. It will be observed that the lists follow the traditional repertory format of bold type, italics and normal type. The gradings indicate the closeness of the link that has been established in a particular case. Those in bold type are what will be referred to as 'leading remedies' in the rest of the text.

The number of remedies that have been positively linked to the nosodes is small compared to the total number that we have available. In part this is due to the creation of new remedies since the bowel nosode work was done, but the main reason has been the therapeutic revolution that has resulted in the widespread use of antibiotics and anti-inflammatory agents, especially steroids. This has meant that the routine obtaining of a meaningful faecal swab is usually no longer easy, and hence the major development work has ceased.

A closer study of the list will reveal that there are chemical patterns in the connections and associations of the remedies, giving a clear link to the disease processes involved with them, and thus another indication that the remedies are truly homeopathic in their nature.

There are many remedies linked to carbon and the carbonates in the associated remedies of Morgan Pure. Proteus is linked to many of the chlorine salts, while iodine is found in many remedies of the Bacillus No. 7 group together with bromine and potassium salts. The Bacillus No. 10 group contains many fluoride remedies. There are also miasmatic connections, which can aid in the selection of the appropriate nosode, although it must be stressed that these are not miasmatic remedies in the same way as the true miasmatic nosodes are. However, it is useful to bear in mind the following broad classifications:

Psora	*Bacillus No. 7*; **Morgan Pure**; *Morgan Gaertner.*
Sycosis	Bacillus No. 7; *Bacillus No. 10*; Coccal Co.; *Dysentery Co.*; *Faecalis*; *Morgan Pure*; *Mutabile*; **Proteus**; **Sycotic Co.**
Syphilis	Bacillus No. 7; *Bacillus No. 10*; *Dysentery Co.*; *Coccal Co.*; **Gaertner Bach.**

Clinical Uses of the Bowel Nosodes

Taking a faecal swab

The therapeutic protocols dependent on a swab are outlined below for the sake of completeness and to assist the basic understanding of the subject. As mentioned above, although theoretically perfectly viable, the effects of conventional medications on the bowel flora have considerably limited their clinical usefulness in the modern age, and the practicality of the procedure is considerably limited by the previous medications (especially antibiotics) that the patient has received. Also the culture procedure required, and the interpretation involved, does not usually form part of standard laboratory services, although there is no reason why the mechanism cannot be set up by special arrangement. The five further uses listed overleaf, which are based on clinical interpretation of the interrelationship outlined above, are practical and useful additions to our repertoire.

Following a swab, various courses of action are possible:

(i) *A positive result, but the NLFB are present at less than 30%.*
Give the appropriate bowel nosode as indicated by the bacteria. The low level of the bacteria indicates that the disease is having a strong influence on the patient, and although some healing reaction is present it is not in the ascendancy. This represents a negative phase in the cycle of the disease. Since the identified bowel nosode is homeopathic to the disease, this is an appropriate remedy selection.

(ii) *A positive result with NLFB present at over 50%.*
Don't give the bowel nosode. If the required remedy is unclear, give the leading remedy of the group indicated by the bacteria, generally in low to moderate potency. This result represents a positive phase, with the body's defences controlling the disease process and having a significant healing effect. All that is needed is some support for that healing reaction. The administration of a bowel nosode at this time may well reverse the ongoing curative process.

(iii) *A positive result with the NLFB present at between 30–50%.*
Either use the remedy in the group most indicated even if it is not a good match. (Use LOW potency.) *Or* give the bowel nosode in LOW potency.
From this single result there is no way of knowing whether the NLFB level is rising, falling or remaining in an unstable balance. A gentle intervention is all that is appropriate in these circumstances.

(iv) *A negative or indeterminate result.*
Use either Merc. Sol. or Tuberculinum if there are any matching symptoms. The exact rationale for this is unclear, but in practice the use of either of these two remedies will often result in a clarifying of the bacteriological picture. As both remedies have a broad action, it may be that their use as appropriate represents a broad enough 'similar' to stimulate the healing reaction.

As remedies in their own right

This is a major use. Each nosode has its own remedy picture, which can be used as the basis of a prescription as with any other remedy. There are also some very clear keynotes to the remedies that can guide their use.

To clear a remedy picture

This may be clearing in the same way as Sulphur and Nux Vomica may be used to clear the system of the effects of conventional medication, thereby allowing the true symptom picture to emerge. Alternatively, if after taking the case no obvious remedy is apparent, a bowel nosode may be used to induce a reaction that results in the emergence of a clearer remedy picture. If all the potential remedies are within the same group, then the related bowel nosode is used. If the choice of remedies is more widely based or very unclear, then the administration of a bowel nosode selected on a strong keynote will often result in a clear indication for the second prescription emerging.

A well selected remedy fails to act, or has only a short duration

The first action in this situation is to check the choice of remedy and the potency at which it was given. If this reappraisal indicates treatment options such as a change of potency or remedy, then these should be implemented. If it is considered that the remedy is correct, and a different potency fails to take the case forward, then the bowel nosode related to the remedy should be considered. Some practitioners will give the bowel nosode as the second prescription and then return to the original remedy if required, possibly at a higher potency.

A variation of employing this remedy-enhancing action of the bowel nosodes is, having selected an appropriate remedy, to give the associated bowel nosode as the first prescription, followed by the selected remedy.

Using an indicated remedy and its related bowel nosode together

In this instance the remedy is used in low potency at a local level and the bowel nosode as a deeper-acting remedy in higher potency. This follows the same pattern as when local and constitutional remedies are used together, with the higher potency being reserved for the constitutional prescription.

To overcome a great sensitivity to a well selected remedy

Occasionally patients are encountered who are so sensitive to a remedy that there is an undesirable reaction. If the choice of remedy is so well matched to the symptoms as to still be indicated, then the related bowel nosode can be used to progress the case without the same problems recurring as were associated with that remedy.

Many sources will advise only using the bowel nosodes in 30c and not repeating within three months. The original workers used them in a range of potencies up to M, and this approach is certainly efficacious in animals. It must be remembered that many of their indications are in chronic disease, and they do need time to act. Although the recommended interval is theoretically correct (Paterson 1949) it should not be regarded as an absolute rule. Remember also that if there is a clearly indicated remedy other than a bowel nosode, then this should be given.

Materia Medica of the Bowel Nosodes

Although some work has been done on provings of the bowel nosodes, the bulk of the knowledge of their pictures comes from clinical experience in both the human and animal spheres. A small amount of work has been done involving faecal counts in dogs and cats suffering from chronic disease, aimed at ascertaining whether the proportions of NLFBs isolated are the same as in humans. Although the number of samples was small, some 300 as opposed to the 12,000 that the Patersons based their figures on, the results indicated a broad similarity with those obtained in the human field (Saxton 1994). Clinical experience also shows a common pattern of response across the species. Although herbivore and ruminant digestions might be expected to give different bacterial patterns, in practice the same clinical indications and results are found to apply.

Morgan Bach

This is a combination of Morgan Pure and Morgan Gaertner. Many of its associated remedies have carbon as a component.

Congestion is the keynote. It acts mainly on the skin and the mucous membranes. There is also a liver involvement.
Mentally there is a restlessness, irritability, tension, and depression. Often a dislike of company.
Conjunctivitis with cysts and styes on the eyelids.
Nasal catarrh with thin clear or white discharge.

Cracks on lips and nose. Dry membranes.

Inflammation of mouth and throat.

Inflammation and congestion of lungs and trachea. Dry cough. Bronchitis, especially attacks that recur every spring.

Desire for fats, sweets and eggs.

Great pain in anterior abdomen. Liver tender to touch. Borborygmi.

Tendency to constipation, but may be looseness in mornings, < eating, fats, eggs.

Foul-smelling motions with some blood and mucus. Motion passed without straining.

Irritation around anus with no obvious cause.

Frequent attacks of cystitis with burning pain. Strong smell to urine when cystitis. Glycosuria.

Stiffness, especially of the shoulders. Pain under the right shoulderblade.

Pustular eruptions on skin. Cracks and eruptions behind ears. Eczema in ears. Cracks around the mouth. Great irritation. Hot red skin. Skin dry and cracked or weeping. Swelling of feet due to much licking.

Skin < heat, washing, teething.

Proteus Bach

Chlorine is a component of many of the associated remedies, and the 'Muriaticums' are well represented in the group. It is rarely needed in the absence of nervous symptoms.

Suddenness is the keynote. Often shows as a 'brain storm' type of symptom, as in epilepsy.

Mentally tense, irritable, The animal may bite suddenly and without warning.

There may be an aetiology of prolonged stress. One area of action linked to this is the adrenal glands.

Many spasms and cramps, with much twitching of muscles.

Abdominal pain with flatulence. Vomiting with blood. Melaena. Bowel upsets connected with digestive allergies.

Irritant vesicles and eruptions on skin with redness.

Likes fats, salt.

Dislikes butter, pork, vegetables.

Eggs can show either a strong liking or aversion.

< wine, storms, heat sun, morning, cold, night.

> resting, eating, in mountains.

Faecalis

Sepia is the main related remedy, and the picture is broadly similar to that.

< fats, sweets

Dysentery Co.

<u>Anticipatory anxiety</u> is the keynote. It is often described in humans as the sort of worry 'that is felt in the solar plexus'. There is thus a difference between this and the continuous stress that is more typical of the Proteus picture.

Fear of people and closed places.

Involuntary twitching of the face.

Chronic indigestion. Nervous diarrhoea. Flatulence. Frequent mucoid stool. Spasm of the pylorus.

Pain in stomach < eating.

Likes sweet food, salt, milk, fat, cheese.

Likes cold drinks but they cause pain in stomach.

Skin dry with dandruff. Crusty eruptions and sticky discharges

Likes heat but is < in stuffy atmosphere.

< 3–6 a.m., crowds.

Gaertner Bach

<u>Malnutrition</u> is the keynote. There is marked loss of weight but the appetite is often good.

Nervous and hypersensitive with a fear of heights.

Otitis externa linked to teething.

Likes eggs, cheese, sweet foods.

Dislikes bread, fish, butter.

Chronic vomiting and diarrhoea. Vomits after eating sweet things. Strong-smelling stool with blood and mucus. Salivation. Cannot digest fats.

Blood and mucus in urine.

Pustular eruptions on head and neck.

Of use in the treatment of worm infestations.

Claimed to be of use in cases where there has been upsets from the overuse of antibiotics.

Bacillus No.7

Related to Iodine, Bromine and Potassium.

Mental and physical fatigue is the keynote. The action is at the neuro-muscular junction.

Pain in the back, especially around the shoulders and neck. Moves slowly. Osteoarthritis in the stifle.

Pain in area of liver with flatulence.

Dislikes fats.

< Cold, damp, draughts, starting to move.

> Heat, rest.

Mutabile

Changeability is the keynote.

There is often an alteration of symptoms, especially involving the skin and another body system.

Metastasis in neoplasia.

Recurrent or sub-acute cystitis.

Sycotic Co.

Irritability is the keynote. This applies on both the mental and physical levels.

Thick yellow discharges.

Conjunctivitis. Photophobia.

Cough < 2–3 a.m. Will cough until sick.

Pain in lumbar and sacral regions. Muscular pain. Exostoses.

Pain in kidneys with strong-smelling urine.

Skin eruptions following vaccination. Vesicular and pustular eruptions. Erythema. Warts and cysts.

Likes fats, cheese, sweets, milk, salt.

Dislikes eggs, potato, tomato, vegetables.

< Cold, damp, eggs, onions, night, first movement.

> Seaside, heat, prolonged movement.

Coccal Co.

Associated with septic states. Low-grade persistent infections.

Care must be exercised to ensure that only short courses are given. Three doses at twelve-hour intervals is the ideal.

Bacillus No 10

Loss of appetite.

Spongy bleeding gums.

Loose motions passed in morning.

Irritation around anus and tenderness around base of tail.

Flat warts mainly on the feet.

Pain in thighs and stifles, especially the left.

Cough with difficult expectoration < morning.

Uterine discharges smell of fish.

Great liking for fried fish and chocolate.

Dislikes eggs and bread.

The Bowel Nosodes and their Associated Remedies

Morgan Pure

Alumina, Baryta Carb., Calc. Carb., Calc. Fluor., Calc. Sil.,
Calc. Sulph., Carbo Veg., Carbo Sulph., Causticum, Digitalis,
Ferrum Carb., *Graphites*, Hepar Sulph., Kali Bich., Kali Carb.,
Kali Sulph., Lycopodium, Mag. Carb., *Medorrhinum*, Nat. Carb.,
Nat. Sulph., Nux Vom., Petroleum, *Psorinum*, Pulsatilla, Rhus Tox.,
Sepia, Silica, **Sulphur**, Thuja, Tuberculinum.

Morgan Gaertner

Calc. Carb., Chelidonium, Chenopodium, Graphites,
Helleborus Niger, Hepar Sulph., Kali Bich., *Lachesis*, **Lycopodium**,
Merc. Sulph., Nat. Mur., Nux Vom., Pulsatilla, Sanguinaria, Sepia,
Silica, Sulphur, Taraxacum.

Proteus

Ammonium Mur., Aurum Mur., Apis Mel., Baryta Mur., Borax,
Calc. Mur., Cholesterin, Conium, Cuprum Met., Ferrum Mur., Ignatia,
Kali Mur., Mag. Mur., Muric Acid, **Nat. Mur.**, Secale, Sepia.

Mutabile

Ferrum Phos., Kali Sulph., **Pulsatilla**.

Gaertner Bach

Ars. Alb., Bacillinum, Cadmium Met., Calc. Fluor.,
Calc. Hypophosphorosa, Calc. Phos., Calc. Sil., Ferrum Phos.,
Kali Phos., **Merc. Viv.**, Nat. Fluor., Nat. Phos., Nat. Sil., **Phosphorus**,
Phytolacca, Pulsatilla, **Silica**, Syphilinum, Tuberculinum, Zinc Phos.

Dysentery Co.

Anacardium, Argent. Nit., **Ars. Alb.**, Cadmium Met., China Ars.,
China Off., Kalmia, Pulsatilla, Tuberculinum, Veratrum Alb.,
Veratrum Vir.

Bacillus No. 7

Ars. Iod., *Bromium*, Calc. Iod., Ferrum Iod., **Iodum**, Kali Bich.,
Kali Brom., **Kali Carb.**, *Kali Iod.*, Kali Nit., Merc. Iod., Nat. Iod.

Faecalis

Sepia, Anacardium.

Sycotic Co.

Antimony Tart., Bacillinum, Cadmium Met., Ferrum Met., Nat.
Sulph., Nit. Ac., Rhus Tox., *Thuja*.

Bacillus No. 10

Calc. Fluor.

Coccal Co.

Tuberculinum.

Bowel Nosodes in Relation to Modern Bacteriology

The original classification involved the use of four sugars – lactose,
glucose, saccharose and dulcitol. All, or most, were of course non-
lactose fermenters, but the exact clinical classification was dependent
on their reaction to the other three sugars.

The faecal swab was initially cultured on MacConkey agar for 18
hours in order to separate the gram-positive bacteria. The colonies of
non-lactose fermenters are then incubated for a further 18 hours and the
resulting colonies added to individual sugar solutions to determine their
reactions.

Each of the bowel nosodes contain a number of bacterial strains within the clinical classification. Some of the clinical entities have no definite bacterial connection. The known groupings are essentially as below.

Morgan Pure

Morganella morganii, Proteus mirabilis, Aeromonas salmonicida, Salmonella subgenus IV, *Edwardsiella tarda, Escherichia blattae, Hafnia alvei.*

Morgan Gaertner

Salmonella paratyphi A, *S. subgenus 2 & 3, Salmonella cholersuis.*

B. Proteus

Edwardsiella hoshinae, Edwardsiella tarda, biogroup 1, Obesumbacterium proteus, biogroup 2, Proteus myxofaciens, Proteus penneri, Proteus vulgaris, biogroup 2.

Dysentery Co.

Shigella dysenteriae, Shigella flexneri, Shigella boydii, Salmonella, Gallinarum, Salmonella typhisus.

Sycotic Co.

Streptoctococcus faecalis, Acinetobacter calcoaeticus lwoffii.

Bacillus No. 7

Citrobacter koseri, Enterobacter cloacae.

B. Mutabile

Morganella morganii, Salmonella subgenus 3.

B. Faecalis

Alcaligenes faecalis.

Coccal Co.

A number of gram-positive bowel cocci.

References

Agrawal, Y.R. (1995) *A Treatise on Bowel Nosodes*. Delhi: Vijay Publications.

Alexander, M. (1988) Re-identifying the bowel nosodes. *British Homeopathic Journal* **77**(2), 67-71.

Bach, E. (1933) The rediscovery of psora. *British Homeopathic Journal* April.

Bickley, A. (2003) Using the bowel nosodes. *The American Homeopath* **9**, 34-39.

Cummings, S. (1978) History and development of the bowel nosodes. *Journal of Homeopathic Practice* **1**(2), 78-90.

Cummings, S. (1988) The bowel nosodes. Bacteriology and preparation. *British Homeopathic Journal* **77**(2), 78-81.

Feldman, M. (1996) *Repertory of the Bowel Nosodes*. New Delhi: B. Jain Publishers.

Julian, O.A. (1995) *Intestinal Nosodes of Bach-Paterson*. New Delhi: B. Jain Publishers.

Paterson, J. (1929) The potentised drug and its action on the bowel flora. *British Homeopathic Journal* **19**.

Paterson, J. (1933) Sycosis and Sycotic Co. *British Homeopathic Journal* **23**, April, p. 160.

Paterson, J. (1936) The role of the bowel flora in chronic disease. *Proceedings of the British Homeopathic Society*, March. Published in the *British Homeopathic Journal*, April.

Paterson, J. (1947) Homeopathic philosophy brought up to date. *Proceedings of the Faculty of Homeopathy Annual Assembly* **25**, June.

Paterson, J. (1949) The Bowel Nosodes. *Proceedings of the International Homeopathic League*, August 1949, Lyon, France. Published in the *British Homeopathic Journal* **40**, 3 July 1950. Available as a booklet published by A. Nelson & Co., London.

Saxton, J.G.G. (1994) Bowel nosodes in animals. *Proceedings of the AVHMA Congress*, Orlando, Florida.

Wheeler, C.E. and Bach, E. (1925) Chronic disease – a working hypothesis. Indian edition published 1987. New Delhi: B. Jain Publishers.

Chapter 14

Vaccination – The Homeopathic Perspective

The Place of Vaccination in Modern Medicine

Vaccination has achieved much for both human and animal health and is justifiably and widely regarded as one of the great success stories of modern preventative medicine. It is credited with the control, and in some cases the elimination, of many major killer diseases in both the human and veterinary fields. From these successes the concept is being extended to encompass disease of all degrees of severity, on the premise that the procedure can do little harm and that its benefits for the majority far outweigh the very occasional adverse reaction.

There are a number of assumptions here which need to be considered. The first is that vaccination has been the prime agent in the control of the major epidemic diseases. Although it is undoubtedly a considerable factor in the situation, the role of improving nutrition and hygiene is often minimised, and there is evidence to suggest that significant reductions in the incidence of many diseases had occurred before the development of the relevant vaccine (Chaitow). It has also been assumed that vaccination, apart from the rare individual failure to respond, is generally effective in creating immunity. In fact a number of studies have shown that this is not necessarily true, and there are recorded instances involving both animals and humans that show a higher incidence of disease in vaccinated subjects compared to unvaccinated ones with the same exposure (Day 1987, Tobin 1992, Trollifors 1984). These studies range across a number of conditions and vaccines. There is no doubt that vaccines stimulate a response in the vast majority of individuals who receive them. However, whether it is always an entirely appropriate response in relation to the total dynamics of the immune response is open to question.

The biggest assumption, however, is that vaccines are essentially harmless. If 'harm' is defined as death or the creation of major disability, then the risk/benefit equation is undoubtedly strongly in favour of vaccination. However, side effects of a much wider, if not so lethal, nature as a result of smallpox vaccination were identified at the end of the 19th century (Compton Burnett 1884), and subsequent experience has shown that the pattern is repeated with vaccination against other diseases. If the chronic ill health that can be caused by vaccination is taken into account in addition to the 'killer' side effects, then the risk/benefit ratio is not so clearly in favour of the procedure.

That is not to say that vaccination should not have a definite place in modern therapeutics. Nor can it be denied that there are considerable benefits to be derived from the use of vaccines. But it must be realised that they are powerful agents with potential for great harm as well as good. It is in the indiscriminate use of, and uncritical attitude towards, vaccines that the dangers lie.

Much work is being undertaken to improve vaccines, moving away from the present basis of attenuated or killed antigens to newer products aimed at involvement of the DNA pathways. But all this is generally within the same context that vaccination is a good thing *per se,* and many of the same potential problems will remain, although an increasing number of veterinary surgeons from both the practice and academic fields are questioning the accepted protocols of vaccine use.

From both the homeopathic and conventional points of view, the use of vaccination against non-life-threatening diseases, the so-called 'non-core vaccines, can potentially cause as many problems as it solves. Even when their use has some justification, the nature of the body's reaction must be borne in mind. A proper and responsible use of vaccination must always be employed, supported where appropriate by homeopathic measures.

Immunological and Homeopathic Considerations

The parameters used to measure immune response in the clinical situation are mainly based on blood sampling. Some doubts are now being raised about the adequacy of this approach as employed in practice, as the fuller and more accurate laboratory tests are not generally available to the majority of practitioners. Reliance is placed on the one single parameter of antibody assessment, which is known not to mirror the complete picture of the immune response. Techniques involving challenge are also available for measuring the efficacy of vaccines, but these are based on trials that are generally ethically unacceptable. Also, while these may provide information about the vaccine's performance overall, they are not practical for measuring the immune status of an individual. The recognised way of doing this is to test the individual's serum for specific antibodies, with the criterion being an adequate level of circulating antibody. The other changes in the composition of the blood associated with the immune response are not usually considered in the clinical context.

Work with distemper vaccine in dogs, based on all these parameters, has shown that the initial effect of vaccination is to reduce the immune response (Phillips 1989). This lasts for up to three days and is then followed by a compensatory increase in activity. The ultimate presence of antibody is then taken to be evidence of an adequate immune response, with the total amount of antibody present being the only criterion. This is then taken further and the continuing presence of circulating antibody is regarded as proof of continuing immunity. Whilst this is true, the opposite inference – that loss of circulating antibody implies total loss of immunity – is not necessarily correct. Trial work has shown that successful response to challenge to distemper in dogs has occurred in animals with titres considered well below the level required for protection (Coyne 2001).

The total immune response of the body involves more than just changes in the blood constituents. There is also an involvement of the endocrine system, with the thyroid gland being particularly affected. Also, by injecting vaccines directly into the body, the immune response at local tissue and cell level of the natural routes of infection is not activated. In the course of a natural infection these latter are the first parts of the system to be involved, with the systemic response only being activated to the degree that the local defences are overcome. A normal *balanced* response to challenge involves both local and systemic involvement *in that order.* The local cellular activity may be regarded as having the function of priming and alerting the potentially greater systemic elements to the need to respond. That response, when it comes, is thus a measured activity appropriate to the challenge.

By contrast, when an antigen is injected directly into the body, the systemic part of the immune system is unprepared and its reaction therefore likely to be more extreme. It may be that the shock to the system thus caused is why there is the initial reduction in immune response following systemic vaccination.

While the production of antibodies is certainly evidence of an immune response, it is not necessarily true that the continuing presence of circulating antibodies is essential for the mounting of a successful

165

defence to field challenge. Once immunity has been established, even if circulating antibody levels have fallen, in the face of challenge they can be restored in less than the 10–14 days required for the initial response. The lymphocytes will retain a memory of the antigen/antibody reaction that has occurred and an appropriate response to subsequent challenge will be made within days. The memory may or may not be lifelong, and may vary with individual infections.

However, a successful response to challenge may involve either a cell-mediated or a humoral response, or both, and if it is primarily the former then antibody levels may not be that important. Thus reliance on circulating antibodies as the sole criterion of immunity will have the effect of underestimating its true level.

In the wild state, of course, there is likely to be continuous challenge, which maintains the antibodies at an appropriate level. But the local tissues of the body will always meet that challenge first. Even in those cases where infection occurs via a bite or other infected wound there is an associated local immune system response before the systemic involvement. Paragraph 186 of the *Organon* states that 'maladies of any import whatsoever, which have been inflicted on the body from without, draw the entire living organism into sympathy.'

All so-called local reactions will always have an associated systemic involvement. In Chapter 2 it was shown that homeopathic remedies work most effectively when administered via a membranous surface, usually the mouth. It has also been established that homeopathy can act by stimulating the immune system. This further emphasises the importance of following the natural routes. From the above it follows that vaccines which are designed to follow the natural route of infection will be potentially less harmful than those given by injection.

So far the considerations have been of active immunity, but the phenomenon of passive immunity also has implications in respect of vaccination. This is generally regarded as being for the primary purpose of preventing the deaths of the young from disease, and is undoubtedly an important consideration. But an immature immune system, having to cope with the challenge of a severe acute infection, is likely to react in an unbalanced way and may be damaged, even if the animal survives. Concerns have been expressed over the effect of multiple vaccinations over a short time scale on immature immune systems via interference with the development of T-cells (Jeffreys 2001). Therefore, an equally important function of passive immunity is *to prevent the immature system from having to cope with a major challenge.*

In the general application of this to vaccination, what is important is not primarily the presence or otherwise of maternal antibodies, but the age by which, in the normal course of events, such antibodies would have waned. This represents the age at which the body has matured enough to mount its own response to challenge without itself becoming damaged. Also, in nature, where there is a background field challenge, this will be met continuously as the maternal antibody level wanes, and thus there will be a gradual change over between passive and active immunity, without there being at any stage the massive challenge represented by vaccination. In domestication, where there may not be adequate initial levels of maternal antibodies, early vaccination can represent a severe shock to the system.

Studies in Japanese children have shown significant reductions in the incidence of cot deaths following changing the age of DPT (diphtheria, whooping cough and tetanus) vaccination from 5 months to 24 months. Post-mortem findings in many cases of cot death fit the pattern of the Non-Specific Stress Syndrome as defined by Hans Selye (Scheibner 1993). The preliminary results of an ongoing survey of Italian Spinones showed a similar trend with 26.6% of animals vaccinated before 10 weeks exhibiting reactions compared with 17.6% in those receiving their first vaccine after 10 weeks (Coombe 1998).

The final factor that must be considered is the use of polyvalent vaccines. While the logistical advantages of this are considerable, the practice may not be in the best interests of the recipient. In Chapter 3 it was shown that the body deals with only one similar disease at a time, and that this concept is at the heart of the dynamics of the homeopathic response. The effect of injecting multiple agents into the body therefore opens up the prospect of unexpected and undesirable reactions. It has been shown that the immune response to one antigen can be compromised by the presence of another antigen. This is in complete accord with the homeopathic concept mentioned above, where the strongest challenge to the vital force will prevail over lesser challenges.

Since the homeopathic response in general involves the immune system, anything that compromises that system must be regarded with grave suspicion. Vaccination has the potential to damage the system. In some instances this will show as frank disease, in others it will manifest as a more general lowering of response, with implications for the efficacy of other treatments.

One other consideration must be borne in mind. The original work (Jenner, 1749–1823) was based on the concept of using cowpox to prevent smallpox. This is in accord with the homeopathic idea of similars. What is now practised is the use of the active disease agent to provoke a response, which is not using a similar agent but using the same, and this changes the nature of the body's reaction. A vaccine's effect on the body will be, in homeopathic terms, a primary action. Further doses of the same, either from booster vaccination or challenge, will provoke another primary action, and as has been shown (Chapter 4), primary action is what is capable of producing disease. In contrast, challenge by a similar will produce a secondary action, which can be curative.

Although vaccination as currently practised raises serious concerns, some of the worst consequences can be avoided by a few simple precautions. The requirements of the data sheets with regard to only vaccinating healthy animals must be adhered to. Vaccination should not be carried out at times when the animal is under stress of any sort. One obvious stress situation is the young animal, separated from its mother and newly arrived in a strange environment. Time must be allowed for adjustment to this, especially if the animal has been subjected to early weaning, which can pose an additional burden. An equally stressful situation is the female animal in either oestrus or early pregnancy – booster vaccination should be avoided at these times.

Also, the practice of vaccination linked to surgical neutering is to be deplored. A link has been demonstrated between infectious agents and hormone activity in the production of auto-immune disease and this should be remembered in this context.

Another major source of trouble is the primary vaccination of animals before the natural waning of maternal antibodies would have occurred. Much of the current work on vaccines is aimed at creating immunity at an earlier and earlier age. This is achieved by increasing the dose of antigen administered, as it has been shown in dogs that the active immune response in the presence of maternal antibodies is related to the size of the dose (Burtonboy 1991). However, in practice, the exact maternal antibody status of every young animal vaccinated is not known. Thus the system of a young animal with virtually no maternal antibody can potentially receive – in effect – a massive overdose, with corresponding detrimental effects. The usual justification put forward for this practice in companion animals is the 'socialising window' of the young. Although this may be a consideration, a far greater consideration is the long-term health of the animal; no matter what type of vaccine is used, the stress on the system will be greater the younger the animal is.

As will be discussed below, there are ways of achieving the best of both worlds without compromising either.

Booster vaccination is another area that gives rise to abuse. In spite of increasing evidence of the longer-term duration of immunity following vaccination (Bohm et al 2004, Elliott and Thomas 2000, Schultz, Kyle, Squires and Davies 2002, AAHA 2003, Douglas 2004), the protocol of annual boosters is still being widely followed. Indeed, endorsement of this practice, and much of the manufacturers' advice, is still being given on the basis of historically perceived guaranteed minimum immune levels rather than those that are currently proven and realistic. It has been shown that re-vaccination of animals with adequate immune levels does not result in an increase of that immunity (AVMA 2000). It is also common practice to use polyvalent vaccines regardless of the necessity for them. All this results in considerable overuse of vaccines, in spite of the increasing acceptance of the view that unnecessary vaccination should be kept to a minimum (Gaskell 2002). Some veterinary organisations are now recommending that booster vaccinations be given at three-yearly intervals rather than annually (AAHA 2003).

Overexposure of the system to gratuitous challenge as a result of too frequent and too broadly-based use of vaccines is a cause of damage to health in many cases. With the methods now available for determining individual immune status, albeit not completely accurate, the avoidance of this hazard is easy within the practice situation. It is also possible to identify the specific diseases against which immunity requires boosting, thereby allowing the use of a monovalent vaccine as necessary rather than subjecting the body to the stress of a polyvalent product. Another consideration is the administration of a vaccine while an animal is receiving other treatment. Apart from the accepted prohibitions in the data sheets, particular care must be taken to avoid the use of vaccines while the animal is receiving homeopathic treatment. As the body will only deal with the stronger stimulus at any one time, the administration of a new and stronger disease in the form of a vaccine can interfere with the response to the homeopathic remedy, especially if it is being used in low or moderate potency.

Harmful Effects of Vaccination

Homeopathic practitioners recognise a condition known as 'vaccinosis'. This is the clinical entity that results from the abuse of the immune system outlined above. It is a clinical entity in the homeopathic sense, in that it is essentially a functional upset representing a true state of 'dis-ease'. How the upset manifests in an individual varies with the miasmatic inheritance and the challenges to which the animal is exposed.

Vaccinosis predominantly increases the influence of the sycotic miasm in the body, and the picture presented will thus have many prominent features of that miasm's action, such as skin conditions involving excess production, and colitis. There is also a destructive type of activity in normal immune function (e.g. phagocytosis), and abuse of the system can on occasion tip the balance too far in that direction, giving a syphilitic action combined with the increased sycosis. Any predisposition to the syphilitic miasm in the animal will increase this tendency. Thus some auto-immune diseases may fall within the scope of vaccinosis. Letterer-Siwe disease in humans, an aleukaemic reticuloendotheliosis known to be linked to vaccination, is clinically similar to the auto-immune anaemia seen in animals.

Immune Mediated Haemolytic Anaemia has been linked to vaccination with the standard canine vaccines (Duval and Giger 1996), with a definite link to booster vaccination having been given within one month of the disease appearing.

Vaccinosis was initially linked to smallpox vaccination, but this was purely a matter of historical timing. Both theoretical considerations and clinical experience show that the condition is linked to the vaccination process rather than any particular agent.

One observation from the early days of smallpox vaccination is of relevance. The criterion for a successful response to the vaccine was the appearance of a skin reaction. If this was not induced the procedure was usually repeated. It was observed that vaccinosis occurred most frequently and most severely in those cases where the skin reaction did not appear. This finding is of course entirely consistent with Hering's law. The skin reaction, interpreted conventionally as indicating a successful vaccination, indicates the body's throwing out of the challenge it has received onto the skin. The failure of this, from the homeopathic point of view, represents the 'dis-ease' remaining at a deeper level.

The diagnosis of 'vaccinosis' will depend on a number of factors, but two major indicators are an aetiology of 'Never Well Since' and the history of a transient systemic reaction linked to vaccination. However, in many cases it is the inappropriate conventional treatment of such

170

reactions that leads to the establishment of more chronic problems. Acute hypersensitive reactions are easily spotted, but other reactions may show a wider range of symptoms. Acute reactions tend to occur either between 24 to 72 hours after vaccination, whereas more delayed responses are seen between 7 and 45 days (Dodds 1983). Although not completely established, there is also some evidence linking the clinical onset of CDRM in dogs to booster vaccination nine months previously (Canine Health Concern Survey 1997). The possible consequences of vaccination may be summarised as follows.

(i) *A general overstressing and unbalancing of the immune system.*
This is particularly relevant in the case of early primary vaccination, but it is also a factor in connection with booster vaccination. Work in both America and the UK is showing that immunity, as measured by circulating antibody levels, is maintained for much longer than is assumed by the proponents of annual boosting, and that boosting of an animal with adequate protection does not actually result in an increase of that protection. However, because of factors discussed above, repeated unnecessary re-vaccination can act as a stress on the system. Even worse is the practice of repeating the whole vaccination course if the stated date for the booster has been passed.

Blood testing for antibody titres offers a practical way of ensuring that an animal remains protected in line with conventional thought, without the unnecessary risks of blanket boosting. (Antibody levels do not, of course, give any indication of cell mediated immunity.) In the absence of complete immunity, it enables the areas of risk to be identified and boosted by the use of the relevant monovalent vaccine, with less risk to the recipient. Although this is not available for all species at the present time, its extension offers a valuable tool against the abuse of vaccination.

(ii) *Possible triggering of hereditary conditions.*
While the inherited tendency will be present irrespective of vaccination, overuse of vaccines may cause the clinical appearance and/or worsening of such tendencies. The heart problems associated with Cavalier King Charles spaniels may fall into this category. Also, the possibility cannot be ignored that the repeated use of vaccines over the generations may finally effect the genetic code. Models for the mechanism by which this may occur are discussed under 'inheritance of miasms' in Chapter 11.

(iii) *Suppression of 'desirable illness' leads to the consolidation of an inherited miasmatic state.*

Some authorities consider that in the process of development, the meeting and overcoming naturally of non-life-threatening illnesses enables the body to clear itself of undesirable miasmatic influences and re-establish the balance so vital for health (Miles 1992). This is one reason why the use of vaccination should be restricted to the major life-threatening illnesses and not utilised to avoid infections from which recovery is the norm.

(iv) *Suppression of normal development.*

This can result from aggressive early vaccination. Adverse effects on the thyroid gland can interfere with the subsequent growth and functioning of the body (Dodds 1994).

(v) *The creation of an obstacle to cure.*

Even in cases where there is no frank vaccinosis, the influence of vaccination may need to be overcome before a cure can be achieved.

(vi) *The creation of chronic disease.*

Vaccination may be regarded as a suppressive procedure, because by ignoring the superficial body reactions and stimulating an initial response at a deeper level, the establishment of 'dis-ease' is encouraged. This is aggravated by suppressive treatment of the body's attempts to control the challenge.

Ointments or baths are commonly prescribed for puppies being presented for the second vaccination, having developed a skin rash following the first injection. This is obstructing the natural process of coping with challenge, and is exactly the situation as described by Hahnemann in relation to his theory of chronic disease. The miasmatic patterns thus created will affect not only the immediate patient but may be passed down to future generations (Chapter 11).

Treatment of Vaccinosis

One approach to this is to use the nosode associated with the vaccination. It is possible to use a true nosode, which has been prepared from the disease process itself. Alternatively a *pathode* may be used. The source material for this remedy is the vaccine itself, and it has the advantage of containing everything that has been administered in the vaccine. Substances such as thiomersal (mercury) and aluminium may be present in the vaccine, and these have been shown to cause side effects in their own right. Whichever product is employed, it may be used either as an initial remedy, or as an intercurrent treatment if the curative process using other remedies has ceased. It will usually be used in moderate potency (30c) as a short course. Their use can on occasion cause marked reactions, with the vigorous reappearance of old symptoms, and hence care must be taken in selecting this approach.

Remedies that have a strong element of the sycotic miasm in their pictures are also of use in these situations. Two of the strongest sycotic remedies are Thuja and Medorrhinum, and these are of particular use when the vaccinosis is uncomplicated by any major influence from the other miasms. They are thus often the remedies of choice in the acute stage following vaccination. The further chronologically one moves from the vaccination, and the more suppressive (usually conventional) treatment that has been administered, the more the other miasmatic influences will come into play. However, all remedies of use in vaccinosis will have a strong sycotic side to them, and consideration should be given to such as Antimonium Tartaricum, Malandrinum, Mezereum, Silica, Sulphur and Triticum, among others.

The rubrics of 'Ailments from vaccination' and '< Vaccination' may be incorporated into a broader-based consideration of a case, but these should not be used as exclusion rubrics unless there is a very strong aetiological connection. Overconcentration on this aspect will often unduly limit the choice available, and as a result the required remedy in a particular case may not be included. The strong suspicion of a vaccine connection in a case can be incorporated into the process of selecting the appropriate remedy by repertorising using other features of the case, and then considering the need for a sycotic remedy in the assessment of the possible remedy choices produced by the repertorisation.

Use of Nosodes in Relation to Vaccination

In addition to the use discussed above, nosodes have a definite role in the treatment of disease, and a possible one in prevention. They are also sometimes used as an alternative to vaccination, although it can be argued that this is not true homeopathy. The use of nosodes in this way also raises important ethical issues which must be addressed. Many owners who wish to pursue this route are under the impression that the use of nosodes is an established and accepted procedure, and do not realise the essentially (from the conventional point of view) unproven nature of nosodes in this role. It is vital that a full discussion of the pros and cons of both vaccination and nosode use takes place with every client who shows interest in the method. It is also essential that the veterinary surgeon, when considering the possibilities, bears in mind their responsibility always to do the best for the animals under their care, and assesses every case in this light.

Extensive work on the efficacy of nosodes in a preventive role is lacking, but some work has been done. However, it has been concerned more with the use of nosodes for protection when given in the face of challenge rather than with their effectiveness as long-term protective agents following short-term administration. The only trial that has been carried out in the latter context, involving dogs and parvovirus, produced a result strongly against the use of nosodes. Although the result was definite, the numbers involved were small and its results possibly cannot be considered conclusive (Larson, Wynn and Schultz 1996).

However, the principle of nosode use in the presence of challenge has been established in the laboratory (Jonas 1995), and studies in disease situations have shown their effectiveness in dogs (Day 1987, Saxton 1991). A trial involving nosode in the successful treatment and control of bovine mastitis has also been recorded (Day 1986).

It is important to realise that if nosodes are used the aim is protection, not vaccination. Vaccination involves the production of antibodies via a systemic response, and antibodies are attractive as they can be easily and accurately measured. As has been discussed above, whilst it is broadly true that a high antibody level confers immunity, the assumption that immunity is lacking unless such a level is present is not justified, as the levels take no account of cell-based immunity. There is also the important question of quality verses quantity of antibody to be considered in this context. In practice the level of antibodies is generally regarded, albeit erroneously, as the major measure of immunity.

The mode of action of nosodes is not fully understood, and various ideas have been put forward. One is that the effect is at cell level and acts via the stimulation of the opsonins in the body fluids, thereby increasing the phagocytic efficiency of the leucocytes and increasing the resistance of the cell membrane to penetration by viruses. The level of opsonins is known to be increased by both vaccination and homeopathic remedies.

Another view is that nosodes 'shortcut' the normal cell information pathways, creating the memory of the disease in the appropriate cells without actual exposure to any antigen. Conventionally the cell memory is being considered as of prime importance in the timing of booster vaccination, and the mode of action of nosodes may be another aspect of the cell memory phenomenon. Whatever the exact explanation may be, circulating antibodies are not present following the use of nosodes, and hence the conventional measurements and techniques are not valid.

When they are used the dosage is oral, thus following the natural route of infection, and the course of treatment is more protracted than a vaccination regime. Slight differences of opinion exist as to the exact protocol although the potency is usually 30c, and primary protection always follows the pattern of a short intensive course over a few days backed by a more protracted regime of reducing dosage over 2–3 months. 'Booster' courses consist of shorter intensive administration at intervals, depending on the risk assessment. It may, however, be advisable to give nosodes continuously in order to maintain protection.

In addition, it must be remembered that the term 'immunity', as used by the conventional world, is often employed in the sense of the animal never becoming ill in the face of challenge. In fact, nature's requirement is that the animal will recover without any serious long-term consequences. Thus by following a natural route to protection it is possible that there may be a transient mild illness following exposure.

When vaccination is employed, the use of nosodes to mitigate any detrimental effects and prevent the establishment of a vaccinosis is considered by many homeopaths to be to the animal's advantage. The appropriate nosode can be also be used in young animals to bridge the perceived gap in protection before the age of natural waning of the maternal antibodies. A short intensive course begun from three weeks of age enables the vaccination to be delayed until a safer time. As nosodes are thought to stimulate the local cellular response, this approach also has the advantage of priming the systemic response before the injection is given, thus simulating the natural progression that is found in an infective situation.

This priming effect may also be utilised prior to vaccine administration at any age, with the corresponding nosode being given for one or two days immediately before the injection. The requirements of boarding kennels, exhibiting, eventing and similar situations for conventional vaccination can thus be met without the risk of harming the animal. There is also the requirement in some countries for compulsory rabies vaccination, and the ill effects of this can be similarly guarded against.

Even if a vaccine has been administered recently, a nosode can still be used after the event, if thought appropriate, to limit any ill effects. A short course as administered beforehand will be required.

One other technique, that of linking the conventional and homeopathic approaches, must be mentioned. Here a short course of nosode in medium potency is administered immediately prior to the vaccination, followed by a single dose of high potency nosode 48 hours after. This is claimed to prevent harmful effects, plus enhancing the immunity achieved (Elmiger 1998).

It is thus possible to obtain the best of both worlds by combining vaccination and nosodes. Vaccination can be a great boon, but it is necessary to be aware of the possible problems that may arise and know how to counter them.

References

American Animal Hospital Association (2003) Report of Canine Vaccination Task Force. *Journal of AAHA* **39**, March/April.

American Veterinary Medical Association Proceedings (2000).

Bohm, M., Thompson, H. et al. (2004) Serum antibody titres to canine parvovirus, adenovirus and distemper virus in dogs in the UK which had not been vaccinated for at least three years. *Veterinary Record* **154**(15), 10 April.

Burtonboy, S. et al. (1991) Performance of high-titre attenuated canine parvovirus vaccine in pups with maternally derived antibody. *Veterinary Record* **128**, 377-381.

Canine Health Concern Survey, 1997.

Chaitow, L. (1987) *Vaccination and Immunisation. Dangers, Delusions and Alternatives*. Saffron Walden: C.W. Daniel Company.

Cherry, J.D. et al. (1998). Report of the task force on pertussin and pertussin immunization. *Pediatrics* (Suppl.), 939-984.

Compton Burnett, J. (1884) *Vaccinosis and its Cure by Thuja*. Published 1887 by Homeopathic Publishing Co., London. Indian edition published 1992. New Delhi: B. Jain Publishers.

Coombes, A.M. (1998-2003) Independent Italian Spinone Health and Vaccination Survey. Rhayader, Powys, Wales. [Ongoing work]

Coyne, M.J. et al. (2001) Duration of immunity in dogs after vaccination or naturally acquired infection. *Veterinary Record* **149**, 509-515.

Coyne, M.J. et al. (2001) Duration of immunity in cats after vaccination or naturally acquired infection. *Veterinary Record* **149**, 545-548.

Day, C.E.I. (1986) Clinical trials in bovine mastitis using nosodes for prevention. *International Journal of Veterinary Homeopathy* **75**, 15.

Day, C.E.I. (1987) Isopathic prevention of kennel cough – is vaccination justified? *International Journal of Veterinary Homeopathy* **2**, 45-51.

Day, C.E.I. (1998) Vaccination and the immune system – homeopathic implications. *LIGA Conference*, Amsterdam.

Dodds W.J. (1993) Vaccine safety and efficacy revisited. *Veterinary Forum* May.

Dodds, W.J. (1994) Nutritional influences on immune and thyroid function. Paper presented at the *AHVMA Conference*, Orlando, Florida.

Dodds, W.J. (1983) Immune-mediated diseases of the blood. *Advances in Veterinary Science and Comparative Medicine* **27**, 163-196.

Douglas, E. et al. (2004) Duration of serologic response to five viral antigens in dogs. *Journal of the American Veterinary Medical Association* **224**(1), Jan.

Duval, D. and Giger, U. (1996) Vaccine associated immune-mediated haemolytic anaemia in the dog. *Journal of Veterinary International Medicine* **10**, 290-295.

Elliott, M. and Thomas, S. (2000) Vaccination revisited. Antibody titres taken in practice reveal a need to reconsider current vaccination programmes. *British Holistic Veterinary Journal* **1**(2), 23-25.

Elmiger, J. (1998) *Rediscovering Real Medicine*. Shaftesbury: Element Books.

English, J. (1992) The issue of immunisation. *British Homeopathic Journal* **81**, 161-163.

Gaskell, R.M. et al. (2002) Veterinary Products Committee working group report on feline and canine vaccination. *Veterinary Record* **150**, 126-134.

Jeffreys, R. (2001) T cells and vaccination. *Lancet* May, 1451.

Jonas, W.A. et al. (1995) Prophylaxis of tularaemia infection in mice using agitated high dilutions of tularaemia infected tissues. 5th GIRI Meeting, Paris.

Kyle, A. et al. (2002) Serological status and response to vaccination against canine distemper and parvovirus of dogs vaccinated at different intervals. *Journal of Small Animal Practice*, June.

Larson, L., Wynn, S., and Schultz, R.D. (1996) A canine parvovirus nosode study. *Proceedings of 2nd Midwest Holistic Veterinary Conference*, Nov. 2–3.

Miles, M. (1992) *Homeopathy and Human Evolution.* West Wickham: Winter Press.

Neustaedter, R. (1996) *The Vaccine Guide.* Berkeley, CA: North Atlantic Books.

O'Driscoll, C. (1998) *What Vets Don't Tell You About Vaccination.* Derbyshire: Abbeywood Publishing.

Phillips, T.R. et al. (1989) Effects of vaccines on the canine immune system. *Canadian Journal of Veterinary Research* **53**.

Rivera, P.L. (1997) Vaccinations and vaccinosis. *Journal American Holistic Veterinary Medical Association* **16**(1), 19–24.

Saxton, J.G.G. (1988) Vaccination, the hidden enemy. *International Journal of Veterinary Homeopathy* **3**.

Saxton, J.G.G. (1991) Use of canine distemper nosode in disease control. *International Journal of Veterinary Homeopathy* **5**, 8-12.

Scheibner, V. (1993) Vaccination. *The medical assault on the immune system.* Mayborough, Victoria: Australian Print Group. Also at Blackheath, London.

Selye, H. (1978) *The Stress of Life.* Toronto: McGraw-Hill Book Company.

Tizard, I. (1990) Risks associated with use of live vaccines. *Journal of the American Veterinary Medical Association* **196**, 1851-1858.

Tobin, S. (1992) An holistic viewpoint on vaccination. 3rd IAVH Congress, Munster.

Trollifors, B. (1984) *Bordetella pertussis.* Whole cell vaccines. Efficacy and toxicity. *Acta Paediatrica Scandinavica* **73**, 417-425.

PART II: THE PRACTICE

Introduction to Part II

Getting Started

Converting a theoretical knowledge and interest into a practical skill can be both exciting and daunting. The important thing is not to try and achieve too much too soon. Initially, limit prescribing to acute conditions with clear-cut indications for remedies. Not only will this be within the scope of the early knowledge that has been acquired, but also the quicker results will impress and encourage everyone. As greater knowledge of the remedies is built up with study and use, the prescribing base will expand and confidence will grow.

Confidence is important. Not only is the subject new ground for the prescriber, but often also for those around, both colleagues and clients. In spite of the growing demand for complementary treatments there is still much confusion in peoples' minds about the subject, as well as a varying degree of professional scepticism.

The new concepts being introduced can appear somewhat strange to an uncommitted person. The less they are talked about the stranger they will appear, and it is important that all who are affected in any way by the new methods are involved from the beginning. Not only professional colleagues but also nursing colleagues and reception staff must be included. The introduction of a few common remedies into the surgery, and especially the routine of the operating theatre, is a good way of including others as well as benefiting the patients.

Clients are often not aware of the range of information that is required, used as they are to concentrating on the presenting complaint. Events such as aggravations and regression of symptoms can be worrying for them unless the possibilities have been discussed. Colleagues also need to be aware of these situations, especially if they have to deal with worried owners out of hours! In addition, the extra time commitment that homeopathy demands, if it is to be done properly, must be emphasised. This is not only the time required for the initial case taking and assessment, because follow-up consultations can also be lengthier that the conventional equivalent. In some cases the time needed for a cure may well also be greater than the client's expectations. Many people have met homeopathy in the acute situation through self-help and have gained the impression that it is always quick-acting. While this is true in many instances, treatment of chronic disease requires time. One rule of thumb is that for every year a condition has been present, one month of homeopathic treatment will be required. This is, however, only an indicator and should not be quoted as a definite rule. The implications for practice of the time aspects of homeopathy must be addressed openly right at the start, and all the administrative and financial implications considered. There is no reason why income from the practice of homeopathy should be lower than from other therapeutic systems, provided that it is priced realistically. It must be remembered that veterinary surgeons should primarily be selling their skills and knowledge, not their drugs. Homeopathy emphasises this but it is true of all practice.

Remedies may be obtained from a number of homeopathic manufacturers, all of whom operate efficient postal services. Hence although the range of remedies and all their potencies may seem daunting, the stock implications need not be that great initially.

Warning! *Homeopathy can be a lonely road.* Most people step out onto this road isolated within their practices, facing varying degrees of scepticism and indifference. The first counter to this is a stated belief in what you are doing and a willingness to discuss it. The same points will be met many times, from a straight 'What is homeopathy?' to the standard criticisms based on the sacrosanct Avagadro's number and what is perceived as a lack of research. It is helpful to have answers to these approaches thought out before they are made.

Most importantly, do not ignore the 'life support systems' that exist outside the practice. Involvement with a training course provides membership of a group of like-minded colleagues, many coping with the same difficulties, plus access to experienced help and guidance. Beyond that are the various national and international homeopathic organisations, such as the British Association of Homeopathic Veterinary Surgeons (BAHVS) and the International Association for Veterinary Homeopathy (IAVH). Membership of these not only gives clinical help via their publications and email forums, but also moral comfort and support.

Combining Homeopathy and Other Treatments

In one sense the distinction made between conventional and other therapies is a false one. The only truly valid distinction is between good medicine and bad medicine. Good medicine is anything that assists nature in its efforts to cure itself. Conversely, bad medicine is anything that interferes with those efforts.

Viewed in this light the use of antibiotics in acute conditions can be good medicine, as it is aiming to achieve exactly what the body is aiming for via phagocytosis and other defence mechanisms. On the other hand, their long-term use in skin conditions achieves nothing curative and, by controlling the skin symptoms without addressing the underlying problem, becomes suppressive.

The questions that must always be asked are 'What is the aim of the treatment?' 'Is that aim compatible with Nature's way?' 'Will the treatment support the system without hindering the curative effort?' Treatments and approaches that impinge on the immune system must be viewed with the greatest caution, as it is mainly through that system that homeopathy works.

There is nothing intrinsically incompatible between homeopathy and surgery, although homeopathy may question the advisability of certain individual procedures – for example, routine 'lumpectomy'.

The greatest differences in philosophy are in the cause and treatment of chronic disease. Even here, conventional medications and interventions can with advantage be employed alongside homeopathic treatment, provided that the true nature of the disease being addressed is recognised. Replacement therapy and certain forms of surgery, such as the selective removal of malignancies, fall into this group.

As experience and involvement increase, cases will be seen that are on long-term conventional medication. On some occasions these treatments will be counterproductive and need to be stopped before real progress can be made. In others, the conventional medication is part of a delicate balance of control. In all situations any change in conventional medication must be undertaken with caution and care.

Homeopathy and other therapies can be used together to achieve the best results for the patient. The other energy medicines, such as acupuncture, are entirely compatible with homeopathy, although the initial use of acupuncture and homeopathy at the same time may on occasion produce too violent a reaction for the patient's good. This may well be true for any combination of energy-based therapies. Herbalism has numerous benefits and overlaps, although it must be remembered that on occasions its philosophical approach can be the same as conventional medicine, especially when used on a self-help basis.

Schuessler Tissue Salts are commonly used in conjunction with homeopathy as both a basic support for the system and a form of local treatment. These twelve salts were developed by a German homeopath, Dr William Schuessler, between 1873 and 1898. The system is not the same as homeopathy, but is a biochemical system based on pathological considerations and the perceived needs of the body for the correction of mineral imbalances. In order to render the minerals into a suitable therapeutic form, trituration and potentisation are employed in the preparation, using the decimal scale, and the prepared salts correspond to a 6x potency.

Correct nutrition supports any therapy, and assessment of diet should always be part of investigation of a case.

No one system can claim to have a monopoly of healing, and to take the best that all systems have to offer in any situation ensures the best results for the patient.

Ethical Considerations

One of the dangers of involvement with homeopathy is the pressure that arises as a result of some requests for treatment. These may come from colleagues who have seen early successes in acute cases and think there is an opportunity to unload problem cases. Such cases are usually complicated and should not be undertaken until sufficient experience has been gained. The idea that no harm can ever be done with homeopathy is wrong. Reference has already been made to the fact that suppression can be brought about by homeopathy (Chapter 8), and too frequent changing of the remedy can on occasion completely derail a case. Other requests will come from owners and will involve species that are not part of the regular work. These must be resisted unless there is sufficient basic veterinary knowledge of the species to make involvement safe.

The acceptance of referrals both implies and requires experience and expertise, as in all disciplines. When accepting these, the normal standards of care and professional courtesy must be observed. It must be emphasised that the guiding ethos must be that of veterinary surgeons who use homeopathy, not that of being a separate group, and the guidance of the Royal College of Veterinary Surgeons, or similar national bodies, should be followed at all times.

Finally, problems can arise as a result of the easy access of the general public to remedies. Requests will be received, often over the telephone, for advice concerning treatment of an animal for which the owner has either purchased a remedy directly, or has access to supply. The guidance of national regulatory bodies in respect of 'animals under one's care' must be observed in these cases.

The Future of Veterinary Homeopathy

This is bright. Not only is there a steadily growing demand for homeopathy from clients, courses are now available to provide adequate training for the profession. Despite reservations in some quarters there is a growing recognition of its value. A steadily increasing number of veterinary surgeons are obtaining an expertise in it. It can be used at all levels of skill, from specialist to general practitioner, incorporating it as part of a broader therapeutic range. The discipline adds a new and broader dimension to the help that the veterinary surgeon can offer. A wider acceptance of its principles will not only benefit the animal world but also increase the professional satisfaction of those who treat them.

How To Use Part II

This is not intended as a short cut to the correct remedy. Prescribing on the 'cookery book' principle will get results sometimes, in the same way that if a dart is thrown at a board often enough it will finally hit the bull. This part is designed as an instructive guide to prescribing. Each section looks at the various systems from the homeopathic point of view, although there is inevitably some overlap with other streams of veterinary thought. All references in Part II to the repertories are to those based on Kent's work, and which hence broadly follow his layout. *Synthesis* is the main one used in this category. Other repertories, such as the alphabetical one compiled by Murphy, have their place, but in the process of a repertorisation it is important to remain within one system. The remedies discussed in each section do not provide a comprehensive list, and consideration should not be confined to them. Many of them will be among the *polychrests* – those remedies that have such a broad action within the body that they find employment in many situations. The materia medica discussed is solely in relation to the system under consideration and does not attempt to present the full picture. The same remedies will appear in different chapters, and it is hoped that by considering particular aspects as appropriate a more complete picture of the remedy will be built up. Similarly, the lists under 'Other Remedies to Consider' should not be thought of as local remedies to be prescribed on a keynote basis. They all have their own broader pictures, and although aspects of these warrant their mention in relation to particular systems, the whole should always be considered. It will be noted that some remedies appear under more than one heading, and it is by blending all these aspects together that a more complete picture may be obtained. Reference should always be made to the full works on materia medica before selecting a remedy.

Reference

Chapman, J.B. (1973) In: Cogswell, J.W. (ed.) *Dr Schuessler's Bio-chemistry. A Natural Method of Healing.* Wellingborough: Thorsons.

Chapter 15

Surgery and First Aid

General Considerations

There are a number of homeopathic remedies whose pathological symptomatology so closely matches that produced by injuries of various kinds that in such situations they may be prescribed with very little reference to the materia medica; they are therefore generally regarded as 'first aid remedies'. Their application in injury, whether accidentally or surgically inflicted, is a most useful way for a practitioner to become acquainted with the homeopathic method. However, it should be remembered that homeopathic principles still apply; these remedies will therefore only be effective if the symptoms presented in the patient correspond to those described in the materia medica for that remedy. In addition it should be noted that these remedies are often polychrests, and their usefulness in homeopathic therapeutics is not limited to their relevance to first aid situations. A detailed study of their materia medica will reveal their true scope in the sphere of homeopathic medicine. However, one of the great strengths of these remedies is that they can be prescribed on very little information, and often simply a knowledge of the initiating cause of the symptoms is sufficient.

The first aid remedies can be enormously effective and their role in counteracting the effects of injury can literally be lifesaving, so much so that it may be tempting to ignore more conventional forms of therapy. While this may be possible in certain minor situations, in others it is clearly erroneous; such procedures as intravenous fluid therapy, general nursing and the dressing or immobilising of injured limbs are clearly measures which are complementary to homeopathy, and are considered to be just as much a part of homeopathic therapeutics as they are of orthodox practice.

Where the situation is acute, the sooner homeopathic medicine can be instituted the better, and drop doses of a liquid potency administered onto the oral mucosa, or tablets placed under the lip, can be administered by the owner before veterinary attention can be received; an

186

animal can also be treated by the veterinary surgeon on its way to the provision of surgical facilities. Doses may be repeated at regular short intervals with complete safety. Remedies in high potencies such as 1M can be administered at intervals as short as five minutes until the patient stabilises. This may then be followed by lower potencies such as 30c at increasing intervals until complete recovery ensues.

When first aid is required there is rarely time to refer to textbooks such as repertories; for this reason it is recommended that the student of veterinary homeopathy learns thoroughly the indications for the following ten medicines.

Aconitum Napellus

Aconite is for shock, whether induced by physical or emotional trauma. The fear, anxiety and restlessness induced by shock are relieved by Aconitum. The provings describe a full, bounding pulse and tachycardia, but in practice shock which has induced a weak, rapid pulse will also respond to Aconite.

Haemorrhage is sudden and profuse; the blood is bright red.

Similar symptoms of fear and restlessness are seen in animals suffering from a high fever, and this represents the second major indication for Aconitum; administration of Aconite at the first onset of fever, before any pathological changes have appeared, will often bring about rapid recovery.

Symptoms are worse at night, for cold dry winds, light and noise; they are better for open air and rest.

Keynote: Fear.

Apis Mellifica

Apis, made from the honey bee, is indicated wherever there is oedema or other accumulation of fluid. This may be the result of local inflammation, or systemic disease such as cardiac failure or renal disease. Insect stings or other allergic reactions will often respond rapidly, and it can be extremely effective in the treatment of angio-neurotic oedema, or 'hives'. The symptomatology includes the oedematous swellings, heat, pain and erythema one would expect to see with a bee sting, but the homeopathic indications comprise any condition where these signs are present, such as acute arthritis or abscess. There is always amelioration from cold in any form – hence in urticaria the pruritus is ameliorated by cold applications. Compare this with Urtica Urens, where there is aggravation from cold applications.

Apis is a thirstless remedy, and correspondingly there is retention of urine. Apis can therefore be beneficial where oedema of the urogenital tract precludes the free passage of urine, and it is frequently indicated in postparturient animals on that basis.

Any acute allergic reaction, where there is oedema, will benefit from Apis so it should be remembered in cases of hydrothorax and peritonitis as well as those conditions of a more superficial nature which have been mentioned.

Keynote: Oedema.

Arnica Montana

The indication for Arnica is bruising, and its effectiveness in this situation is what has caused Arnica to become the most commonly used homeopathic remedy around the world. It often represents a person's first experience of homeopathy and has certainly been responsible for demonstrating the efficacy of this form of medicine more than any other remedy.

In acute injury it is given at any potency, but generally the higher the better, even 10M, as soon as possible after the event, and as frequently as necessary thereafter. In surgery, it is useful to commence dosage the day before the operation, and during surgery drop doses can be administered sublingually by the anaesthetist. Postsurgically it may be continued at lower potency, e.g. 30c b.i.d. This also applies to dentistry, where the anti-haemorrhagic effect of Arnica makes it so extremely useful. Aural haematomas, especially if surgery is contraindicated, will benefit from Arnica, and postparturient bruising is yet another indication.

The provings include 'bruised feeling', difficulty getting comfortable when lying on hard surfaces, and pain and stiffness of muscles which is relieved on motion. Pain on touch may be so great as to lead to a fear of being touched.

The homeopathic effect of Arnica in bruising reduces pain considerably and it is the authors' experience that when it is used properly, if necessary in conjunction with other homeopathic remedies, it is only in extreme cases that conventional postsurgical analgesia is necessary.

Keynote: Bruising.

Carbo Vegetabilis

The state of collapse is where this remedy proves its value; traumatic shock, septicaemia or hypovolaemia can all precipitate the Carbo Veg. state. There is coldness, air hunger, torpor and cyanosis, and the patient may be bloated. There may be foul-smelling eructations or flatulence. Dyspnoea is ameliorated by sitting up.

Paradoxically to the extreme coldness of the body which Carbo Veg. exhibits, the patient is ameliorated by fanning; similarly, it resents being covered and will attempt to throw blankets off. There may be oozing of dark blood from wounds or any orifice. The pulse is weak to the point of being imperceptible and the patient may tremble or shiver.

The ability to reverse such states of utter collapse has earned Carbo Veg. the epithet of 'corpse reviver'.

Symptoms are worse at night, for cold, and in the open air; they are better for fanning and for eructations.

Keynote: Collapse.

Hypericum Perforatum

Hypericum is for injury to nervous tissue; as such it is of immense value in pain relief, especially in injury to areas rich in nerves such as the skin and extremities such as toes and tail. Given around the time of surgery, pain relief is accompanied by rapid healing of wounds. Pain caused by injury to the spinal cord is also relieved – the provings include pain in the cervical area, made worse by the slightest movement and relieved by bending the head backwards. Convulsions due to concussion of the head or spine also indicate Hypericum, and lacerations of the cornea will benefit.

Keynote: Pain from injury to nerves.

Ledum Palustre

Penetration wounds of soft tissue are the field of action of Ledum. This can include animal bites, insect bites or penetration wounds inflicted by sharp objects such as nails and fragments of glass. In the eye there is haemorrhage, either subconjunctival or intraocular.

The wounds of Ledum are cold and in this context Ledum has a beneficial effect in tetanus, where there is twitching of muscles near the wound.

Sprained hocks are also an indication for Ledum, where there is swelling and bruising causing a characteristic blue discolouration. Ledum pains are relieved by cold applications

Keynote: Puncture wounds.

Hypericum and Ledum have a reputation for aiding in the prevention of tetanus.

Staphysagria

This remedy is for skin wounds, especially those caused by surgery. It is mentioned in the materia medica as being for 'ailments from cuts with sharp objects'. There is great sensitivity of the tissues, and wounds of the orifices are particularly involved. Severe pain after abdominal operations is considerably relieved by Staphysagria.

The mental aspects of this remedy centre round indignation and suppressed anger, and this, coupled with its association with surgery accounts for its indication in any condition, be it cystitis, inflammatory bowel disease, miliary dermatitis or inappropriate urine spraying which follows surgical neutering; 'Never well since neutering' is enough to merit consideration of Staphysagria.

Staphysagria is also indicated in compound fractures.

Symptoms are worse for touch, anger or grief, and better for warmth and rest.

Keynote: Postsurgical pain.

Symphytum Officinale

This medicine is manufactured from comfrey, the folk-name for which is 'bone-set'. This refers to its use in herbalism for aiding in the healing of fractures, and it is here that Symphytum finds its niche in the homeopathic materia medica also. Any damage to bone or periosteum will heal more rapidly with the administration of Symphytum, and it can be invaluable in the treatment of non-union fractures. Given periodically over the healing period of a fracture it will prevent such problems, encouraging swift healing with minimal callus formation.

Injuries to the eye caused by blunt objects also benefit from Symphytum.

When there has been injury to muscles and periosteum, especially around joints, Symphytum will be beneficial, and it can be a useful follow-up to Arnica in this context.

Symptoms are worse for movement, touch and pressure and better for warmth.

Keynote: Injury to bone, cartilage or periosteum.

Ruta Graveolens

Sprains and strains are the realm of Ruta. In particular, tendons and tendon sheaths are affected, though periosteum and cartilages are also mentioned in its materia medica. One of the main indications for Ruta, therefore, is tendinitis, especially of flexor tendons; also tendinitis of the Achilles tendon. Pain on palpation is accompanied by stiffness which improves with motion. Sprains of any joint represent a major area of influence for this remedy and it is therefore indicated in cruciate ligament injuries, so much so that the conservative treatment of these injuries becomes more feasible. If surgery on the joint is performed, Ruta administered pre-and postoperatively will speed up healing and improve recovery times.

Bursitis is also an indication for Ruta.

There is stiffness of the back, which is better for lying on the back and for pressure.

Mentally the patient is weak and lethargic; in humans there is despair.

Symptoms of Ruta are better for warmth, motion and rubbing, and worse for cold, damp and overexertion.

Keynote: Sprains.

It will be noted that the locomotor symptoms of Ruta bear resemblance to those of Rhus Tox. However, Ruta is indicated when the symptoms are more the result of injury or chronic overexertion. There is also some similarity with Arnica and it is therefore common practice in veterinary homeopathy to use a mixture of Rhus Toxicodendron, Ruta Graveolens and Arnica ('RRA') as a first aid remedy in any condition showing symptoms of pain and stiffness which is improved by motion. This can be a useful approach in this situation, as long as the drawbacks to such a local approach and to multiple prescribing are appreciated.

Calendula Officinalis

Calendula is one of the few medicines which are commonly used topically in homeopathy; applied to wounds in the form of a lotion or a cream, it prevents infection, reduces granulation tissue and accelerates healing. It also acts as a haemostatic and can be particularly useful in this field after tooth extraction. Where secondary infection has already occurred, or where there is excess granulation, Calendula acts as a cleansing agent and aids in the resolution of these states. In these cases it is also indicated in potency. It is a useful cleansing agent in otitis externa.

One of the areas where Calendula can be most useful is in the treatment of dehisced surgical skin wounds; application of Calendula cream reduces irritation and speeds healing to such an extent that in all but the most extensive dehiscences, the need for resuturing is obviated.

Lotions are made by diluting the mother tincture in distilled water 1:20; creams are available from homeopathic pharmacies.

Keynote: Open wounds.

Other Remedies to Consider

Calcarea Sulphurica
    Abscesses where pus has found an outlet.
    Pus is thick and yellow

Hamamelis
    Haematomas
    Haemorrhage of dark blood
    Varicosities

Helleborus Niger
    Concussion
    Rolling of the head
    Pupils alternately constricted and dilated

Hepar Sulphuris
    Painful abscesses
    Low potency encourages suppuration, high potency suppresses.
    Slightest touch is painful

Silica
    Chronic suppuration where discharge is thin and watery
    Solar abscesses in cattle
    Aids expulsion of foreign bodies such as grass seeds
    Follows Hepar Sulph. well

Chapter 16

The Upper Respiratory System

General Considerations

Because much of acute respiratory disease is viral in origin, homeopathy represents a form of medicine which can make a marked difference to how veterinary patients of any species experience disease. The severity of the symptoms can be rapidly reduced and the course of the disease curtailed, thus avoiding many of the chronic sequelae so frequently encountered in veterinary practice. If the disease has become chronic, then the improvement in immune response which homeopathy is capable of eliciting can be instrumental in initiating long-term improvements. Even such refractory infections as aspergillosis of the nasal cavity can respond to accurately prescribed homeopathic remedies. The general rules of homeopathic prescribing of course apply, but in such deep-seated chronic infections as aspergillosis, and indeed in some of the cases of chronic sinusitis encountered in cats and horses, specific nosode therapy can be a useful adjunct to more classical homeopathic prescriptions.

The upper respiratory system encompasses several distinct anatomical entities, viz. eye, nose, mouth, throat and lymphatic structures. Often the disease process is reflected in all of these areas; where it is not there is more opportunity for individualisation of the patient, and if symptoms in one part are different from another this represents a 'strange rare and peculiar' which can be of immense value. Euphrasia, for instance, has acrid discharges from the eye and bland discharges from the nose; Allium Cepa has the reverse.

Miasmatic influences are often clearly exhibited in the upper respiratory tract. Psora shows dryness and poor immune response, sycosis exhibits profuse nasal and ocular discharges and benign tumours such as nasal polyps, while Syphilis is responsible for ulcerations and erosions of nasal septa, turbinates and oral mucosa. Thin, bloodstained discharges suggest such erosive processes. Chronic corneal ulceration and keratitis also suggest Syphilis, although refractory ulcerations of the cornea in the absence of vascular reaction

193

suggest Psora. In chronic fungal diseases the combination of granuloma and destruction, and the poor immune response responsible for the infection getting a hold, lead one to consider the tubercular miasm, and much chronic upper respiratory disease generally may be attributed to this miasm, while the cancer miasm is well represented by the nasal and oral tumours which are encountered with ever-increasing frequency in veterinary practice. Chronic or recurrent tonsillitis also suggests the tubercular, or less commonly, the cancer miasm.

Suppression of the discharges which emanate from the upper respiratory tract may well cause the disease to exhibit symptoms at a deeper level; rhinitis may lead to sinusitis, which in turn may lead to lower respiratory disease or other symptoms associated with the miasm. Joint disease has been observed as the consequence of suppression of a sycotic upper respiratory disease. Upper respiratory disease therefore represents a fairly superficial level of disease in an organism and so it represents an opportunity to redress the imbalance in the vital force before deeper levels of disease develop. Nevertheless, there is no doubt that this system can throw up some difficult therapeutic challenges, not least of which is the chronic plasmocytic gingivitis observed in cats. The miasmatic basis of this is debatable; the overreaction of the immune system suggests Sycosis; the ulceration, seen so severely at the fauces, suggests Syphilis and there is argument for a tubercular basis. Whatever the theoretical considerations, this condition often remains refractory to treatment. This is not to say that these patients are incurable, indeed complete cures are observed from time to time, usually following a constitutional prescription. However, in many cases palliation is the best that can be achieved.

As a final note, it is worth remembering that the upper respiratory system is one of the organ systems capable of expressing laterality, and this should be borne in mind when using symptoms from this area.

Major Modalities and Rubrics

As upper respiratory disease can affect so many separate areas, there are frequently a number of symptoms available. Listed below are those considered most useful for accurate homeopathic prescribing:

(i) Nasal discharges; amount, character (acrid or bland), colour, viscosity, presence of blood, and laterality.

(ii) The presence of crusts; stoppage of nose; movement of the alae nasae, with or without respiration.

(iii) Ulcerations of nasal septum, alae nasae or cornea.

(iv) The presence of sneezing and any modalities thereof, such as entering a warm room or going outside into cold air. Is the sneezing in isolated episodes or is it in paroxysms?

(v) Ocular discharges: amount, character, source (e.g. conjunctiva or puncta lacrimalis), involvement of meibomian glands.

(vi) Photophobia. Is this worse with natural or artificial light?

(vii) Swellings of nasal, maxillary or mandibular bones.

(viii) In the mouth; gingivitis, ulceration of the mucosa and exact location thereof, the condition of the teeth, the presence of gingival hyperplasia, epulis or other benign tumours; the presence of malignacy.

(ix) Swelling and pathology of tonsils and local lymph glands.

Other information such as is available by endoscopy and radiography may also prove useful in making a homeopathic prescription and should be sought wherever possible.

Remedies of Major Use

Arsenicum Album

Acrid, burning discharges characterise Arsenicum Album. Watery discharges burn the skin over which they run, and cause ulceration. The conjunctiva is injected, lid margins are red and there is oedema around the eyes, especially of the lower lids. There may be corneal ulceration, though this is not a common feature of the Arsenicum ocular disease; however, there is consistently intense photophobia, particularly for daylight. Similarly, discharges from the nose are acrid and burning and there is violent sneezing. Despite the fact that the discharges are watery the nose may still be obstructed, necessitating mouth breathing. The sense of smell is lost; this may be exhibited in cats by looking for food and then turning away from it. The mouth is dry, but there may be superficial ulcerations of the mucous membranes ('aphthae'). Symptoms are paradoxically improved by warmth in any form, though in acute conditions the head symptoms may actually be ameliorated by cold. All symptoms of Arsenicum are aggravated at the seaside. Periodicity is also marked with Arsenicum, thus symptoms may be aggravated every 7 or 14 days. The animal is either prostrate, its apparent condition being out of proportion to the symptoms, or is anxious and restless, hiding away in the warmest place it can find.

Pulsatilla Nigricans

In contrast to Arsenicum, Pulsatilla has bland discharges; not only that but they are thick and creamy, usually green, but may tend towards white. Pulsatilla is right-sided, so there may be unilateral ocular discharge or at least the right eye may be affected more severely than the left. The eyes also itch so the patient may rub them. Chalazion may occur. The nose, too, produces thick bland creamy discharges which may block the nostrils and, as with Arsenicum, there may be loss of smell. Symptoms are worse in a hot stuffy room and ameliorated by fresh air and gentle exercise. There is also aggravation from lying with the head low; this allows comfort-loving Pulsatilla another excuse for lying with her head on a cushion! Pulsatilla is changeable, so upper respiratory symptoms may vary from day to day or even hour to hour; they may change location or change in severity.

Natrum Muriaticum

Discharges in Natrum Mur. are the colour and consistency of raw egg-white, a characteristic feature of the Natrum Mur. discharges wherever they may be from. Discharges may be clear or slightly opaque, occasionally bordering on white. Usually ocular discharges are bland but equally they can be watery, and although there may be tear staining, burning of the skin is not common. Nasal discharge has the same characteristics and there is much sneezing; indeed, if the first symptom of disease is sneezing, Natrum Mur. is frequently effective in preventing disease from progressing any further. Loss of smell and taste are again possibilities. Tears may flow from coughing. Natrum Mur. symptoms are worse for lying down, at 10 a.m., at the seaside and in a warm room; they are better in the open air. The animal generally prefers to be alone and resents any form of consolation.

Silica

Silica is the chronic of Pulsatilla; in other words, if an animal whose acute symptomatology corresponds to that of Pulsatilla is not treated, it may progress into a Silica state. Similarly, a patient who suffers from repeated episodes of acute disease which respond to Pulsatilla should benefit in the long term from Silica. There are many such relationships in the materia medica; Calc. Carb., for instance, is the chronic of Belladonna. This being so, the mental symptoms of Silica bear some resemblance to those of Pulsatilla, in being yielding and timid. In contrast, however, Silica is extremely chilly, can be obstinate and wishes to be warmly wrapped up. Silica is particularly valuable in chronic disease, especially of a suppurative kind, therefore in the context of upper respiratory disease there is chronic watery or purulent ocular discharge, and the cornea may be ulcerated to the point of descemetocoele. Hypopyon may also be present, and there may be iridocyclitis or keratitis with opacity of the cornea. Photophobia is worse in the daylight. The lachrymal duct and sac may also be inflamed or blocked.

The nose may crack, and there is chronic watery or purulent discharge which forms dry hard crusts; when these are removed the tissue underneath bleeds. The nose may be completely obstructed and the septum may be eroded to the extent of perforation.

Tonsils may be chronically enlarged, as are the associated submandibular and cervical lymph glands; however, these glands are cold and painless. Symptoms are worse for cold conditions, damp, uncovering and in the open air; also for pressure.

Mercurius Solubilis

Mercury causes ulcerations and is destructive of tissues. The syphilitic nature of Mercurius shows itself in a preponderance of eye symptoms: there is a burning acrid yellow discharge, sometimes even with blood. The eye itself exhibits keratitis, iritis and hypopyon, and ulceration with intense photophobia which here is worse for glare, especially that from an open fire. Blepharospasm may be evident.

The nose may be ulcerated, both inside and on the nostrils, and ulceration of the mucous membranes of the mouth result in profuse salivation with a foetid smell. Sometimes the saliva is bloodstained. Sneezing may cause epistaxis, as may coughing. Gums, too, may bleed. Tonsils are enlarged and may be ulcerated; lymph glands painfully swollen.

The Mercurius patient is generally hurried and may be aggressive, though in illness he may be dull and lethargic. The patient is extremely thirsty for large quantities of water. Symptoms are worse in extremes of heat or cold, changing weather and damp cold, and there is aggravation between sunset and sunrise. They are better for rest.

Other Remedies to Consider

Aconitum Napellus
   High fever; early stages of equine or feline influenza
   Red swollen lids
   Hot watery discharges

Argentum Nitricum
   Purulent ophthalmia
   Ulceration and photophobia
   Discharges yellow

Gelsemium
   Fever with lethargy
   Thin acrid watery discharges
   Sneezing, especially in the early morning

Hydrastis
   Thick yellow discharges
   Ophthalmia
   Sinusitis

Phosphorus
   Blood-streaked nasal discharges
   Sudden epistaxis
   Gingivitis with bleeding

Chapter 17

The Lower Respiratory System

General Considerations

Consideration of the embryological development of the respiratory system, plus the role of the system in relation to survival and Hering's law, will give a guide as to the true nature of many of the conditions that are met with. Conventionally we recognise laryngitis, bronchitis, pneumonia, pleurisy, asthma, emphysema, neoplasia and the secondary complications of cardiac disease. From the homeopathic point of view, in many cases these will be only the descriptions of the end product of disease rather than of the disease itself. Thus the classification discussed in Chapter 7 is applicable. However, in the case of the respiratory system there is an additional consideration in connection with suppression. Because of the common embryonic derivation of the tissues from endoderm, there is in many cases a strong link with the effects of suppressive medication on the skin. Thus we see the 'asthma/eczema seesaw', where the alleviation of symptoms in the one system is mirrored by a worsening in the other, and this can be observed in all species. It must always be borne in mind that the manifestations of this link are not confined to asthma. COPD in horses is another condition that will often show this pattern.

Many of the respiratory conditions that are seen in practice will be part of a chronic disease picture and a constitutional approach will thus be indicated. However, there are also many instances of primary acute situations seen in the system, and prescribing here will be based on more local and keynote symptoms, although any mental or general symptoms available should be used.

Another factor is the inter-relationship with the heart. Although this is recognised and considered in the conventional approach, the resulting prescription(s) will be based on the reductionist concept of two separate systems that closely influence each other. It cannot be emphasised too strongly that homeopathically this separation is counterproductive. In any assessment of the respiratory system, signs relating to the heart should be included as part of the overall picture.

Horses appear to be prone to the development of respiratory malfunction as a major part of their vaccinosis picture.

Major Modalities and Rubrics

Changes involving movement and exercise tolerance are of great importance, as not only are they closely related to the conditions encountered, but can be easily and accurately observed. Descriptions of types of cough should be viewed with a degree of caution, the evidence of the prescriber's own ears being in many cases the only reliable basis. The results of auscultation, when linked to that, will provide useful information. Any laterality revealed is important. There can on occasion be marked differences as to which areas of the lungs are affected and which side they are on. This may correlate with a laterality of nasal discharges.

Atmosphere and temperature must be investigated. Due allowance must be made for those species where respiratory exchange forms the major part of the heat exchange mechanism. Cases occur where heat has no influence but a stuffy or oppressive atmosphere does. Such cases will be neutral about heat, or even seeking it, but will be > outside. Cases that are > outside in winter may be showing a true heat modality.

This situation can be seen in an animal that is a Pulsatilla constitutional type.

Although time is a useful modality it may often be subject to the owner's lifestyle. A seasonal connection can also be useful, especially in chronic cases.

Position of standing or lying should also be considered. This may be linked to laterality, but there can be changes in position linked to the ease of respiration.

The colour, consistency and ease of expectoration of any discharges must be noted.

In the repertory, the chapter on Respiration contains rubrics in connection with the functioning of the lungs. Physical signs, plus some symptoms, will be found under Chest. The Larynx/Trachea section should be utilised and the chapters on Cough and Expectoration should not be neglected. The Generals chapter is relevant with regard to modalities and preferences.

Remedies of Major Use

Arsenicum Album

With Arsenicum there is a marked aggravation between 12 midnight and 2 a.m. It is a chilly remedy with a great liking for heat. It is generally > heat, and conversely < cold. When ill the slightest exertion gives prostration. There is often both a physical and mental restlessness in the patient. Respiration is rapid, with wheezing, < lying down. The cough is dry, with the head held low and the neck stretched forward. Discharges are thin and acrid; may be grey in colour. Respiratory signs often show after the suppression of dry scaly skin symptoms.

Lycopodium

A marked feature of the remedy is an aggravation between 4 and 8 p.m. There is a right-sided laterality generally, but in the respiratory system this usually shows as conditions starting on the right side and then spreading to also involve the left. It is > heat with a definite dislike of, and aggravation from, wind.

There is a deep dry cough with difficulty breathing, as if the system were blocked.

Discharges are watery. There is a flaring fan-like motion of the nostrils which is not synchronised with the breathing, but this may be difficult to see. Although conditions tend to be slow in onset, it has a role in the treatment of pneumonia. A useful guide to the remedy is a difference in temperature between the feet, especially involving the front legs. The right side is often warmer than the left.

Phosphorus

With respiratory problems the breathing is rapid, with an irregularity that can give the impression of inspiration being cut off before it is finished. The cough is hard and dry.

In normal circumstances there is a large thirst for cold water. Although this is still there in illness, swallowing more than a small quantity at a time may be impossible due to the breathing difficulties. Because of the generally destructive nature of the remedy and its tendency to bleeding, there is often some blood in the discharges, which are otherwise yellow/green. There is a suddenness about the onset of Phosphorus conditions. The pulse is weak and rapid. It is an important remedy in pneumonia. There is often a strong laterality present, with the left lung being markedly more affected than the right; cases will be seen where only the left lung is involved, with the right remaining clear.

Sulphur

This is a major remedy in all spheres. Because of its position as Hahnemann's great anti-psoric remedy, it is not surprising that one of the guiding features is that of respiratory symptoms appearing after suppression of eruptions. Although most Sulphur constitutional types dislike heat, the more reliable indications are < heat and a desire for open air. These may also be seen as local modalities, indicating the possible use of Sulphur as an intercurrent remedy in cases involving other constitutional types. There is general shortness of breath, with loose cough and mucus in the lungs. The pleurae are often involved.

Tuberculinum

There are various forms of Tuberculinum available. Tuberculinum Bovinum is probably most widely used in veterinary work, and is discussed in Chapter 12.

Tuberculinum Aviare (from chicken) is also available. The other two common forms are Tuberculinum Koch (from culture of human bacillus) and Bacillinum (from human sputum). Of these, Bacillinum is often of great use where the respiratory system is primarily involved.

The connection with the tubercular diathesis, or tendency towards a particular disease syndrome, makes this an important remedy. Although cattle are the species most affected by this in the animal sphere, its use in other species must not be forgotten. There is a changeability and restlessness about the remedy that is different to that of either Pulsatilla or Arsenicum Album. In Tuberculinum there is a *dissatisfaction with the present lot or situation*. Horses may continually try to escape from fields, dogs easily become bored with the same food, and dairy cattle may continually go into every stall other than their own. On the physical level there can be a constant changing of symptoms, plus the failure of well-selected remedies to act. Emaciation in spite of good appetite is a feature. Respiratory symptoms appear quickly and easily in response to the slightest challenge. Breathing is difficult, even in open air. Skin symptoms are dry with intense irritation.

Ammonium Carbonicum

The Ammonium salts generally have a marked action on the respiratory system, but the carbonate has most involvement with the lungs. It is a right-sided remedy. The breathing is slow and laboured. There is an accumulation of mucus in the chest, although little is brought up. The cough is dry and mainly at night. Signs are < for exertion and warmth and > cold air. Lung conditions are seen associated with weakness in the heart.

The pulse is rapid and hypostatic congestion occurs. There is a thin nasal discharge.

Its uses include pulmonary oedema, allergic conditions, pneumonia, emphysema, and chronic bronchitis.

Antimonium Tartaricum

Respiratory signs and symptoms are very marked in this remedy, and this represents its main area of use. It acts on all mucous membranes, producing large amounts of mucus, and all systems may be affected. There is often much mucus in the chest and rattling can be heard on auscultation. However, the animal has great difficulty in raising it, and the cough is non-productive. The effort causes much salivation and may lead on to vomiting. The vomit contains mucus from the stomach. Breathing is rapid and shallow. Together with the mucus in the lungs this gives an inability to obtain enough oxygen, and there is often a degree of cyanosis. The dog or cat must sit up to breathe, and the horse or ruminant will stand with the neck extended. The pulse is weak and rapid. The effort involved in breathing, together with the lack of oxygen, gives great weakness. Those animals that sweat will do so. It is useful in pneumonia, emphysema and pulmonary oedema.

Bryonia

Bryonia primarily affects serous surfaces, and hence the pleura are its main seat of respiratory action. A major guiding feature in all cases is < movement and a great desire to avoid all movement. The Bryonia patient does not want to be disturbed in any way, and can become bad-tempered if it is. There is also a local modality of > firm pressure. Animals needing Bryonia will therefore remain as still as possible, leaning against a hard surface, as there is also a desire to sit up. The breathing is shallow, to minimise movement. The low oxygen intake that this produces means that there is a periodic desire to take a deep breath. The attempt to do this results in a dry cough. Dryness and heat are other features of the Bryonia picture. The mucous membranes are dry to the touch and there is a great desire for large quantities of water. The breath is hot.

Drosera Rotundifolia

Serous membranes are again affected. There is rapid shallow breathing with a dry spasmodic cough. It is < at night especially after midnight, and on lying down, > in the open air. The spasmodic cough can lead to attacks of choking with cyanosis. The pulse is rapid and irregular. The larynx is sensitive to touch in humans and this will sometimes also be seen in animals. In people it is used to treat whooping cough and tuberculosis, and in dogs it has a particular role in the treatment of kennel cough, together with pneumonia and pleurisy in all species.

Other Remedies to Consider

Beryllium Metallicum
   < movement
   Dyspnoea
   Dry cough

Ferrum Phosphoricum
   Moderate fever
   Haemorrhages from nose and lungs
   Spasmodic cough

Hypericum
   Asthma and allergic reactions involving the lungs
   Harsh cough
   Much mucus is brought up, which gives relief

Lobelia Inflata
   Shallow breathing
   Cough is < slight exertion but > rapid motion
   Emphysema

Morgan Bach
   Inflammatory congestion of the throat and lungs (kennel cough)
   Cough < in morning
   Bronchitis especially in winter and spring

Chapter 18

The Digestive System

General Considerations

It must always be remembered that the lining of the digestive system is in fact an external surface of the body, and that it is continuous with the skin. As well as the ingestion and absorbing of food, the system has an elimination function beyond the mere expulsion of digestive waste. The mouth is also an integral part of the immune system, not only because of the lymphoid tissue closely associated with it, but also because stimulation of the mucosal surfaces is the first trigger to the cellular immune response.

The whole state of the mouth, including the teeth, is therefore the first consideration. Although homeopathy can help in restoring and maintaining oral health, conventional dental procedures should never be rejected.

The next consideration is the role of diarrhoea in disease. Even acute diarrhoea is an attempt by the body to heal itself. Many apparently acute bowel conditions are part of a chronic disease picture. The onset of diarrhoea is often a part of a healing action. It may represent either one facet of the exteriorisation of a condition in accordance with Hering's law, or a regression of symptoms. Hence any rush to counteract it, especially with conventional agents – but also with homeopathic remedies used in a palliative manner – may be counterproductive. Suppression of a regressing symptomology can reverse the direction that a case is moving in, and halt the curative process. There will, of course, be situations where diarrhoea must be treated, but the above considerations must always be borne in mind.

In the context of chronic disease, there are some remedies (e.g. Antimony Crudum, Croton Tiglium) which have a distinct connection between skin and bowel symptoms. In view of the developmental and physical connection between the two systems this is not surprising, but when using them Hering's law must always be remembered. The direction of cure will always be towards the skin, with normal bowel activity being restored and with the appearance of skin symptoms.

205

Thus even in acute conditions the choice of remedy will ideally involve consideration of other aspects of the animal.

Diarrhoea is not the only symptom that is shown by the lower bowel, although it may be the one most often presented. Constipation can be as significant homeopathically.

The modalities of an acute bowel episode can be very useful in determining the underlying constitutional picture, and some miasmatic indications may be obtained from the symptomatology. Pain*less* bowel conditions are indicative of psora; pain*ful* ones indicate sycosis.

The matter of intestinal parasites must be considered. A truly healthy animal will have an increased natural resilience to these infestations, but many are not in that happy state. It is therefore inevitable that situations will arise where these problems have to be addressed. While some homeopathic remedies have an action against worms it is doubtful if these should be relied on entirely, especially in group situations. Intensive management systems on farms are particularly inappropriate situations in which to rely on vermicidal remedies.

The action of remedies is twofold. There is some vermicidal activity but in addition the general condition is improved, allowing the animal to 'live with the problem' more easily. Thus, in a group, the whole burden may rise unnoticed until crash point arrives. Homeopathic remedies may be able to maintain a worm-free environment, but in view of the above, plus the ethical and public health aspects, conventional worming should be considered in clinical situations.

Major Modalities and Rubrics

A time modality and any changes in general symptoms can be especially useful in acute prescribing for animals about whom little is known, and the timing of any symptoms in relation to eating in general or any particular foodstuffs is a vital part of the case-taking.

Around the mouth, note should be taken of the colour, heat and dryness of the membranes. Care must be taken to differentiate between salivation and mucus production. Much is made of changes to the appearance of the tongue in the human field, and the organ has both secretory and excretory roles among its functions. However, with a few exceptions the authors have not found these signs to be particularly useful in animal work. The swelling of the tongue associated with Mercury is perhaps the most useful, while the 'mapping' of the tongue as part of the Natrum Mur. picture can be helpful.

Where pain is present, the investigation of movement, heat and pressure modalities is valuable.

The consistency, colour, frequency, volume and odour of the stool are important.

Also the presence of blood and/or mucus, and the difficulty or ease of passing the motion, together with any indications of pain or irritation. If tenesmus is reported, it is necessary to ascertain its exact timing in relation to the passage of the motion.

Flatulence is regularly encountered, and note should be taken of its location, any pain associated with it, and its routes of passage. The normal digestive physiology of the various species must be borne in mind when assessing the significance of this symptom. If passage is via the anus it may involve the simultaneous passage of faeces.

The repertory chapters on Mouth, Teeth, Throat, Stomach, Abdomen, Rectum and Stool contain the bulk of the rubrics. It should be noted that in newer versions of the repertory all rubrics relating to food and drink are in Generalities. Modalities relating to eating and drinking will also be found in Generalities.

Remedies of Major Use

Arsenicum Album

This is one of our major polychrests, and there is a marked action on the bowel. There may be an aetiology of eating rotten food, especially fruit. Both vomiting and diarrhoea are seen. The diarrhoea is watery, and is passed either without effort or with only moderate tenesmus. Occasionally it is passed in an explosive spurt. In some cases, unless it is seen to be passed, its appearance may be confused with urine. Blood may be present in both the vomit and diarrhoea, and mucus in the stool. There is a strong smell of putrefaction.

There is prostration out of proportion to the severity of the upset, and a marked desire for heat can appear, even in animals who normally prefer a cool environment. The thirst is for small quantities of water at a time, but the total intake may be higher than normal.

Although the pains of Arsenicum are burning they are relieved by heat. There will often be a restlessness due to pain, and in appropriate species a hot water bottle applied to the abdomen will give relief. The general feature of aggravation around midnight is often seen in relation to bowel conditions.

The liver and spleen can be enlarged and tender to the touch, and ascites due to liver involvement is seen. There is a cessation of rumination in appropriate species.

Mercurius Solubilis, Mercurius Corrosivus

Mercury affects every part of the body, the effect being primarily destructive. In the present context there is an action on the digestive and lymphatic glands. The two remedies largely differ only in degree, the Corrosivus being the more intense. The Mercurius animal reacts to extremes of any sort. Symptoms are generally < from sunset to sunrise. The action on glands and mucous membranes produces excessive secretions. In the mouth there is profuse salivation, with inflammation and ulceration giving bleeding and a foul smell. The gums become soft and swollen. If there is vomiting it is bile-coloured and may contain blood. There is intense tenesmus, with diarrhoea that contains much blood and mucus. It has a strong smell and is usually green in colour, but may be grey and watery. There is abdominal pain linked to the diarrhoea, and the liver is tender to the touch. Blood in the urine often accompanies the diarrhoea. There is a thirst for large quantities of water at a time. Discharges are generally yellow-green in colour and acrid.

Nux Vomica

Here there is a bad-tempered nervous animal with a low pain threshold. There is chilliness and a great liking for heat. It is a useful remedy where there has been much previous medication. The keynote aetiology is overindulgence. It has a major action on the stomach and liver. Conditions are < mornings, overeating, rich food, pressure and movement. Flatulence is a marked feature, causing abdominal pain in spite of some being passed. The carnivores will vomit. There is normally a tendency towards constipation with ineffectual straining. Where diarrhoea does occur it contains blood and mucus, with the first part being soft and the last part becoming firmer.

Another part of the picture is spasm. Together with the flatulence this makes it a major remedy for colic in horses and the keynote of overindulgence gives it a role in some cases of laminitis. At the other end of the scale it is useful where there is flatulence as a result of inactivity in the bowels.

Phosphorus

This is another remedy that is linked to destruction of tissues. The liver and pancreas are both affected by it. There is a desire for salt and spicy foods, with a great thirst for cold liquids. There is also a dislike of, and aggravation from, warm food and drink, and this, coupled with the desire for cold things, may show in domestic pets as a willingness to eat food straight from the refrigerator, or to drink straight from the tap. In carnivores, water – and to a lesser extent food – will be vomited back within five to ten minutes of swallowing. There is great prostration. The gums are ulcerated, with swelling of the tonsils and mucus in the mouth. Liver and spleen may be enlarged and tender to the touch. Diarrhoea is pale and watery and there is abdominal pain, even though the motion is passed easily. Haemorrhage occurs easily and all discharges and excretions are likely to contain blood in significant amounts. The stool contains mucus. Fatty motions are associated with pancreatic disease. Conditions are usually of sudden onset. Although there is a liking for cold food and drink, other conditions are generally < cold. There is also a general worsening at night, often with a marked fear of the dark.

Parvovirus in the dog is a strong indication, due to the bleeding that is often seen in the condition.

Phosphorus has been helpful in rectal prolapse and also in cases of vomiting following anaesthesia.

Veratrum Album

Copious, Cold, and Collapse are the keynotes of Veratrum in relation to the digestive system. There is excessive vomiting and copious watery stool that may contain blood.

The vomiting and the diarrhoea may occur together. Non-productive retching can continue after the stomach has been emptied. There is great coldness of the whole body and a desire to be covered. (This is in contrast to Camphor, which has the same collapse and coldness but which will attempt to move away from coverings and heat.)

There is an increased thirst for cold water, which is vomited immediately. There is abdominal pain with flatulence and much straining to pass the motion. The evacuation can be forceful. Symptoms are < movement and cold drinks and > warmth and lying still.

Other Remedies to Consider

Carbo Vegetabilis
    Much retained flatulence and borborygmi
    Passage of wind does not give relief
    Foetid diarrhoea with straining
    < eating

China (Cinchona Officinalis)
    Debility from loss of fluids
    Flatulence with relief by passing it
    Colic > arching the spine forward (doubling up)
    Watery diarrhoea. Foul smelling and containing undigested food
    < eating fruit and drinking milk

Colocynthis
    Sudden onset
    Great abdominal pain coming in waves. > arching spine forward
    Yellow, watery diarrhoea passed with spluttering flatus
    < eating and drinking. > movement

Iris Versicolor
    Action on the liver and pancreas
    Loss of appetite
    Vomiting of bile
    Watery diarrhoea linked to pain over the liver

Magnesium Phosphoricum
    Flatulent and spasmodic colic. Constant passing of flatus
    Watery diarrhoea
    Desires very cold drinks
    > for warmth and pressure

Chapter 19

The Stomach and Liver

General Considerations

These two organs are included in the same chapter not only because they are anatomically related, but also because malfunction of the liver is generally reflected in symptomatology of the stomach.

The stomach and liver suffer from all of the major miasmatic patterns. For instance, poor liver function may be psoric, hepatitis may be sycotic, cirrhosis or gastric ulceration syphilitic and carcinoma of either organ may be due to cancer miasm. Banerjea suggests that duodenal ulcer is tuberculinic.

The liver of course is the hub of the metabolism, and is the one organ above any other which suffers the onslaught of toxins ingested or introduced parenterally in the form of medicaments. Preservatives such as are frequently found in dried commercial foods, NSAIDs and chemical parasiticides are but a few examples of compounds which have to be metabolised by the liver, with the inevitable consequences. Furthermore, feeding concentrates to cattle and horses lays stress on the liver.

It is not surprising, then, that Nux Vomica, one of the most important liver remedies, is also a remedy whose state is induced by toxic overload, and this serves once again to emphasise the role of diet in the homeopathic management of such cases.

Symptoms associated with liver dysfunction can affect virtually any other organ system, but homeopathic physicians have been highly observant in this field, so collecting all the subtle changes evident in the patient may well direct the prescriber towards one of the major liver remedies without actually having made a definitive diagnosis. One such example is the dryness and desquamation of the skin which in homeopathy, and herbalism, is considered to be an indication of a poor liver function, possibly evident before pathological changes bring about the biochemical changes detectable by routine blood analysis. Progression of this pathology leads to the hepatocutaneous syndrome now recognised by orthodox veterinary medicine.

Having said this, as the liver and stomach are organs not easily accessible to palpation, reliance on haematology and blood bio-chemistry, ultrasound, X-radiography, biopsy or endoscopy may well be necessary for a definitive diagnosis, and the importance of this cannot be overemphasised. Symptomatology itself will not be enough to accurately prescribe for a dog with a gastric carcinoma, or a horse with ragwort poisoning, and elucidating the cause of ascites consequent on a cirrhotic liver will be essential in correctly managing the case.

Nevertheless, the liver is an organ which has legendary powers of regeneration, and patients with severe liver disease are often cap-able of making remarkable recovery when properly treated with homeopathy.

Finally, many patients presented for homeopathic medicine generally are in a state of liver dysfunction consequent on their previous orthodox management. It is often advisable to initiate treatment with organ remedies in low potency with a view to redressing this imbalance, before proceeding on to more specific management of the presenting complaint. The state of the liver may in these circumstances be con-sidered to be an obstacle to cure, and far better response will be obtained with subsequent homeopathic treatment if this problem is dealt with first.

Major Modalities and Rubrics

The stomach has its own chapter in the repertory, whereas liver symptoms are mainly found in the Abdomen section. Vomiting is a symptom which has major importance in homeopathic prescribing, as there are so many ways in which the pattern can vary. The type of vomit is important, be it watery, frothy, bloody, mucoid or of bile or food, the latter whether undigested or not. Similarly, time modalities are useful, especially those relative to the time of ingestion. A symptom which is common in humans is that of regurgitation of acid from the stomach ('heartburn'). This is described in the repertory as 'waterbrash' and is sometimes reported by dog owners.

The rubrics for Nausea can also be used if the required symptom cannot be found under Vomiting.

Pain can often be elicited in conditions of the stomach and liver, and its location can be a useful pointer to remedies, as it may be referred to areas other than those normally expected from an orthodox point of view.

Swelling of the liver is a sub-rubric of Abdomen; swelling, and there is also a rubric of 'Abdomen; liver; enlarged'.

Jaundice is found under 'Skin; discoloration; yellow'. Petechial haemorrhages are also found under 'Skin', this time under 'Eruptions; petechiae'.

Ascites is found under 'Abdomen; dropsy', and oedema ('Edema') of the abdomen is a sub-rubric of 'Dropsy', but also occurs in the other chapters, such as Extremities.

Remedies of Major Use

Arsenicum Album

With Arsenicum there is vomiting of fluids and food immediately after eating. In addition there may be vomiting with simultaneous passage of a diarrhoeic stool. Vomiting of bile is also a symptom of this remedy, and the nausea may be so great that vomiting may occur at the smell or sight of food. As cold in any form aggravates, warm food or water may remain in the stomach; but the thirst for small quantities of water at frequent intervals, so characteristic of this remedy, easily leads to the cycle of drinking and vomiting frequently seen in viral infections of dogs and cats, be it panleucopaenia, parvovirus or infectious hepatitis.

Swelling of the abdomen occurs with ascites and an enlarged and painful liver and spleen. There may be jaundice.

The Arsenicum aggravation after midnight, with restlessness and chilliness, is once again in evidence.

Phosphorus

The sudden onset of so many of Phosphorus' symptoms is readily evident in the vomiting, acute liver pain and petechial haemorrhages of acute hepatitis. Undigested food is vomited 'when warmed in the stomach', which seems to be between five and ten minutes after ingestion. Vomit may also contain bright red blood. The stool may be clay-coloured and there may be jaundice. Phosphorus is one of the main remedies indicated for postoperative vomiting.

Nux Vomica

The Nux Vomica picture is induced by overeating; in humans the desire for spicy foods along with copious quantities of stimulants such as alcohol and coffee make Nux the pre-eminent remedy for hangovers. A similar effect on the canine liver can be induced by a diet of processed foods rich in additives and long courses of such hepatotoxic agents as NSAIDs. Food is vomited undigested, or there may be vomiting of bile. There may be unproductive vomiting and soreness of abdominal walls, and pain on palpation of the stomach. There may be pain in the stomach some time after eating, especially in the morning, and Nux is indicated in gastric ulceration. There is chilliness and constipation, and the patient has a bad temper so is likely to bite or kick at the slightest provocation.

Chelidonium Majus

Jaundice is prominent with Chelidonium. There is swelling of the liver and pain, but the pain is characteristically referred to the back, under the caudal angle of the scapula, particularly on the right side. Pain in the stomach is temporarily relieved by eating, especially hot food and drink.

The tongue is swollen, showing the imprint of the teeth, and the alae nasae may flap independent of respiration. Stools are yellow, pasty, clay-coloured and may resemble sheep-dung. There is a lack of thirst and a desire for cool air, and the patient is drowsy and languid.

Chelidonium's almost specific effect on the liver has resulted in its being used as an organ-specific remedy. In low potency, Chelidonium is likely to have a beneficial effect on almost any liver disease.

Lycopodium

Lycopodium is one of the more flatulent remedies in the materia medica. This is reflected in the bloating of the stomach, which creates the feeling of fullness after eating associated with this remedy. The result is that an animal which seems to be hungry will take a few mouthfuls of food and then walk away. Paradoxically, and therefore of great prescribing importance, hunger is greatest at night. Loss of weight despite a good appetite is a feature of Lycopodium, and this is seen with the cirrhosis of the liver which may respond to it. Other symptoms of liver dysfunction include ascites and sensitivity of the liver, especially the right lobe, and vomiting of bile.

Other Remedies to Consider

Carduus Marianus
   Jaundice
   Cirrhosis with ascites
   Pain in liver < lying on left hand side

Hydrastis Canadensis
  Weakness, cachexia
  Cancer of stomach or liver; gastric ulceration
  Constipation; stools covered or mixed with mucus

Kali Carbonicum
  Nocturnal vomiting of food
  Jaundice and ascites
  Patient is obese, chilly and sensitive to noise
  Symptoms < 2-4 a.m.

Magnesium Muriaticum
  Hepatitis; painful, enlarged liver. Pain < lying on right-hand side
  Dry, whitish or pale stool
  Milk aggravates

Natrum Sulphuricum
  Acute and chronic hepatitis
  Desire to lie on right side with legs curled up
  Diarrhoea with flatulence
  All symptoms aggravated by damp in any form

Reference

Banerjea, S.K. (1993) *Miasmatic Diagnosis.* New Delhi: B. Jain Publishers.

Chapter 20

The Urinary System

General Considerations

As so much of the function of the urinary system involves the elimination of waste products, disease in this area has serious consequences. It thus represents a deep level of imbalance in the vital force. Conversely, any major change in the strength of the vital force may be reflected in increased efficiency of the urinary system, and it is not uncommon to see urine output increase as a result of a successful homeopathic prescription. What might be more alarming is the increase in waste products that may ensue; cellular debris and inorganic matter in the form of crystalluria may be voided in the urine as part of the improvement of renal function so instigated, and it is well to be aware of this.

It is the sycotic miasm which predominates in this sphere, and suppression of a more superficial sycotic disease may well lead to urinary symptoms. Similarly, repeated suppression of a recurring cystitis, either by long-term antibiotic or – worse – corticosteroids or other anti-inflammatory therapy, will eventually lead to renal failure. It may be interesting to compare the orthodox explanations for this progression with the homeopathic philosophy which predicts it. Orthodox medicine sees this as a natural progression of the disease, or else as the result of side effects of the medication, whereas homeopathy considers the deepening disease process as a predictable consequence of suppressive drug therapy. Sycosis is also exhibited in the form of calculus formation – this is considered to be an overreaction of the organism over and above the normal excretion of mineral waste. Crystalluria itself is seen as simply another symptom of imbalance of the vital force, to be taken along with all the other symptoms presented in the total picture, and not necessarily the cause of the urinary frequency and haematuria which may accompany the crystalluria. As such, controlling the crystalluria by dietary means does nothing to address the fundamental energetic imbalance underlying it, and therefore can at best be palliative. Taken logically, if the vital force is denied this form of expression then it may find another way and produce other symptoms, and these may well be on a deeper level again. This is not to negate the value of prescription diets in causing the dissolution of calculi already existing, or in preventing their recurrence while other therapeutic measures are put in place, but the long-term reliance on such diets is contrary to homeopathic philosophy and in this light should be viewed critically. On the other hand, the role of diet in the development of Feline Lower Urinary Tract Disease (FLUTD) is well recognised and failure to address this area constitutes an obstacle to cure. FLUTD has its basis firmly rooted in the sycotic miasm and any attempt to treat this condition will be more successful if this is borne in mind.

Still on the subject of calculi, it is generally accepted in the field of veterinary homeopathy that calculus formation in the urinary tract is associated with a defective hepatic function; most of the remedies which are recommended in such cases are also recognised as having a major effect on the liver.

With renal failure, it is worth noting that whether the disease is acute or chronic, much success may be found in treating this condition homeopathically in dogs and cats. Improvement of blood parameters may be seen, and even animals which have been given a hopeless prognosis on the basis of massive rises in blood urea and creatinine have recovered after homeopathic treatment. Once again, dietary changes may be beneficial but the authors' experience is that in small animals a reduction in protein levels, along with an improvement in quality by more reliance on eggs, dairy products and fish, is all that is needed.

In considering miasmatic influences, the destructive processes which typify much renal disease show the mark of syphilis, though the tubercular miasm may also be involved. The latter is often evidenced by wasting despite increased appetite.

Urinary incontinence can also be treated very successfully with homeopathy; it is useful to ascertain whether the underlying cause is hormonal, emotional or physical, although it must be borne in mind that there is an emotional aspect to all disease and that the key to success in this field, as with all homeopathic medicine, is in getting to grips with the mental and emotional state of the patient.

Major Modalities and Rubrics

The repertory contains separate chapters on the Kidneys, Bladder, Urethra and Urine, but while all these sections may yield useful rubrics it is perhaps those dealing with the bladder and urine which are most commonly appropriate to the symptoms observed in disorders of this system.

Where bladder disease is concerned the most easily observable sign is that of frequency. The degree of this needs to be noted, along with any other modalities such as the effects of heat or cold and time on the pattern of micturition. 'Urging' is a rubric which describes the straining observed in cystitis. Characteristics of the urine need to be noted: quantity, colour, presence of blood, mucus or visible sand or calculi. The smell of the urine is also important. Laboratory examination for albumin, pH and specific gravity, and microscopic examination of the sediment for casts and crystals will also yield valuable information, and chemical analysis of calculi can be of importance. All these parameters are covered in the repertory, under the sections of Bladder or Urine.

Symptoms of renal failure such as increased thirst and vomiting must be investigated critically; pattern of thirst and character of vomit can be vital in choosing homeopathic medicines and the time modalities in particular can be of paramount importance. These rubrics are found in the 'Stomach' chapter.

It is worth remembering that renal pain may be referred to the back, and in these circumstances it is relevant to use the symptoms of pain in the chapter on 'Back'. However, where pain is evident on direct palpation of the kidneys, or where pain can be inferred from the posture of the animal, the rubric 'Kidney; pain' should be used.

With incontinence, rubrics such as 'Bladder; urination; involuntary' and 'dribbling' are useful, as are modalities such as 'during sleep' and 'first sleep'. Movement modalities such as 'rising from seat' or 'while walking' can be useful.

Finally a reminder that the pathology itself is unlikely to be the determining factor in choosing the correct homeopathic remedy; whether the animal is suffering from glomerulonephritis, interstitial nephritis, amyloidosis or FLUTD, success will depend on accurate analysis of the urinary symptoms presented by the patient, in conjunction with careful elucidation of the concomitant, general, and mental symptoms which mark out that animal as an individual.

Remedies of Major Use

Arsenicum Album

This medicine is of major importance in the treatment of renal failure, especially in cats. The increased thirst is exhibited in the characteristic pattern of wanting small quantities often. Vomiting of food occurs immediately after eating and vomiting of bile is common, particularly after midnight. Urine may be profuse but may also be scanty and burning and the colour may be dark, even being described as like 'cow dung water'. Albumin is present. Ulceration of the mouth occurs and the renal failure is often accompanied by dryness and desquamation of the skin, producing large quantities of white dandruff.

Natrum Muriaticum

Thirst in Natrum Mur. is extreme; large quantities and often. Urine is copious, pale, and of low specific gravity. However, there may be some embarrassment at passing urine 'in public', so in cats these very private individuals may conceal their polyuria by always going outside, thus avoiding the litter tray. There is weight loss, particularly around the neck, despite a ravenous appetite, and the ion imbalance of chronic renal failure is reflected in Natrum Mur.'s craving for salty foods such as crisps or salted fish. The albuminuria of renal failure leads to ascites and fluid retention, strong features in the Natrum Mur. picture. Polyuria may lead to involuntary urination especially on coughing, sneezing or walking. Natrum Mur. is the remedy most likely to produce a 'clearing out' of the kidneys, and large quantities of cloudy urine may occasionally be passed for a short time after treatment commences. The 'egg-white' discharges of Natrum Mur. are represented by a discharge of clear mucus from the urethra after micturition. The mouth has aphthae and gingivitis and the coat is greasy.

Phosphorus

Phosphorus has thirst for large quantities of cold water; in cats and dogs this is exhibited by a preference to drink from puddles, fish ponds, plant pot holders, bathroom taps or toilet bowls. If there is vomiting this occurs five to ten minutes after ingestion; food therefore returns undigested. Like Natrum Mur., Phosphorus craves fish and salt, and again there is weight loss despite a ravenous appetite. Phosphorus however bleeds, so urine is often bloody; in cystitis there may be bloody urine with no other signs of disease, and the gingivitis of renal failure is exhibited as a thin red line along the gingival margin in an otherwise clean mouth; the gums bleed when touched. Urine contains albumin and phosphate crystals or calculi. Biochemistry reveals high levels of phosphorus in the blood, and in common with the previous two remedies there is anaemia. Although most frequently indicated in chronic renal failure, Phosphorus is probably the most commonly indicated medicine in acute nephritis; hence the pain in the area of the kidneys which does not allow the patient to lie on his back.

Mercurius Solubilis

Being one of the most 'thirsty' remedies, and being associated with so much tissue destruction, it is not surprising that Merc. Sol. is frequently indicated in renal disease. There is extreme thirst for cold drinks, which may be vomited some time later – despite the wetness of the Mercurius mouth. The mouth is ulcerated and there is copious, foul-smelling, bloody saliva, often with periodontal disease and even pyorrhoea and apical abscess. Urine is albuminous, often with large amounts of blood, and in cystitis there is frequent tenesmus after urination. Following the suppurative nature of Mercurius there may be large amounts of mucus and pus in the urine. The urine is also acrid, and wherever it touches the body it irritates the skin. For some reason, Mercurius seems to be more frequently indicated in renal failure of dogs than of cats. Symptoms are worse at night.

Cantharis

Given the close match of the symptom picture of Cantharis to most cases of acute cystitis, it is perhaps to be expected that it should come to be seen as a specific in this condition. From a classical view point this is inherently erroneous, as the homeopath always seeks to match the prescription to the individual; nevertheless Cantharis remains one of the most effective and easily prescribed medicines in our homeopathic armoury. The symptoms of Cantharis can easily be visualised by considering that the source of the remedy is the Spanish Fly, whose legendary aphrodisiac properties result from a low-grade irritation of the urethra. Larger dosage induces a severe burning sensation which affects the whole length of the urinary tract. Thus there are frequent attempts at micturition which are either completely unproductive or result in the passage of only a few drops of urine, sometimes with a little blood. Symptoms are worse for touch, and better for rubbing – in this context this seems to equate with licking in animals. The affected cat therefore runs to the litter tray, cries out and strains hard to produce no more than a few drops of blood-tinged urine, then licks vigorously at its penis or vulva. Symptoms are also relieved by warmth.

Cantharis may also be indicated in acute renal failure; here there is acute sensitivity of the area over the kidneys in addition to the symptoms already described.

Other Remedies to Consider

Berberis
Renal colic; pain extends along ureter
Back pain associated with renal disease (especially evident in horses)
Urine turbid with red sediment; oxalate crystals
Chronic cystitis, pyelonephritis

Causticum
Bladder paralysis; retention of urine
Recurrent cystitis; follows Cantharis well
Urinary incontinence < walking, coughing

Equisetum
Tenesmus
Passage of large quantities of urine
Incontinence, especially where no other cause except habit

Hydrangea
Cystic calculi in sheep and goats

Pulsatilla
Haematuria
Intermittent cystitis
Involuntary urination especially in the young; < lying on the back, from excitement

Sarsaparilla
Severe pain at close of urination
Sediment of white sand – FLUTD
Passes blood or white acrid material at close of urination

Chapter 21

The Female Genital System

General Considerations

This is perhaps the system in the animal body that is most abused and exploited by man. One danger is that because some procedures have become so standard, it is easy to forget just how much stress and functional abnormality is being produced by them.

In the food-producing animals the manipulation is towards increasing reproductive activity. Although this may appear to be broadly in line with nature it can create its own problems, associated with the hormonal procedures employed to increase reproductive activity and the general stress of over-production. This is still an interference with the normal reproductive cycles, and it can lead to problems within the system due to the resulting upset to the natural balance and process. But in general terms the problems created are not so severe as those associated with the frank suppression of all reproductive function that is perpetrated in small animals. Also, as mentioned in Chapter 5, the problems in farmed animals are largely submerged and concealed by the commercial requirements that drive the management systems. That does not mean, however, that they are not created.

While over-breeding is the main abuse in the commercial sphere, in the companion animals it is more often under-breeding that can lead to problems. The key to understanding this from the homeopathic point of view is that the genital system (in both sexes) is a major site of the physiological activity involving the creation of new tissue. Indeed, it could be argued that the normal physiological function of cell and tissue creation is the 'raison d'être' of the reproductive system. Thus when the normal physiological functions within the reproductive system are upset, and as a result a miasmatic pattern is created, the natural tendency is for this influence to be the sycotic miasm. But as has been seen, the normal physiological functioning is always in balance with the other physiological forces that are active within the body. Anything that interferes with that balance, or prevents its re-establishment, creates the potential for clinical problems.

Social requirements mean that female companion animals are inevitably going to be kept in reproductively abnormal conditions. The various techniques employed to achieve this all have their strengths and weaknesses in general terms, but it is necessary to be aware of the homeopathic implications of the procedures.

Surgical neutering is the commonest single method of control. The complete removal of the system does indeed preclude the subsequent development of pathology within it, but it also means that the body has one less natural outlet when attempting to deal with disease. The process of cure requires such outlets, and if the natural ones are blocked, then others will be found.

A sycotic trait, with its characteristic overproduction of tissues and discharges, in a sexually entire patient, may find its predominant expression via the reproductive system; but if this has been removed, that may result in the appearance of sycotic manifestations in other systems. Also, in a neutered animal, the hormonal balance of the body is without the appropriate influence of the levels of hormones associated with overt sexual function.

There is an ongoing debate regarding the ideal age for neutering. Neutering before puberty results in a balance being created, as the animal matures, which takes account of the changed situation. Neutering after puberty means that the body has to attempt to re-create a balance after the existing one has been disturbed. It could be considered that such a neutered animal can never attain a true balance, and that the significance of this increases in proportion to the number of seasons that have occurred prior to surgery.

Sexually the hormonal balance revolves around the triad of pituitary–adrenals–gonads. Following the removal of the one leg of this balanced relationship, it is the pituitary that is most affected in the necessary adjustment because of its central role in the hormonal regulation of the whole body.

As indicated above, in entire animals there may be the appearance of clinical conditions in the reproductive system as part of a deeper chronic picture. Many of the conventional approaches to these conditions will be extremely suppressive, and this must always be remembered when deciding on a course of action in cases that come to homeopathy following conventional treatment.

Chemical methods of reproductive control involving conventional hormonal preparations are suppressive in the extreme and should be avoided at all costs, as should their use in clinical situations. Continuous routine use of these methods is particularly hazardous. Because of the vital role of reproduction in the continuation of the species, and the resulting emphasis on the creation of new tissue as the prime function of the system, continual blocking of that function produces major upsets. It is an important concept in homeopathy that suppression of the body's attempts to deal with disease will drive the process inward to deeper levels and systems. Suppression of the normal functions of a vital system can result in malfunction within the system, which may result in pathology.

It must not be forgotten that the mammary glands are an integral part of the genital system, although in normal circumstances the increases here are of secretion rather than tissue. However, the considerations discussed above involve these glands as much as the rest of the system, and it is interesting to note that many of the problems occurring in humans are being seen in the mammary glands, with the consequent appearance of cystic and neoplastic conditions. In cattle the use of prostaglandins and other similar agents may have an influence on the incidence of mastitis in a herd.

Since homeopathy works by assisting and stimulating the natural responses of the body, it will be realised that the concept of contraception is alien to the philosophy.

Using the principle that sarcodes in high potency will inhibit glandular function, some degree of control of oestrus may be possible. Other remedies that are of use in nymphomania, such as Murex, have been advocated as these may control excessive behaviour. It is however of limited effectiveness and is not to be advised – the approach is basically as suppressive as using any chemical agent, both of them being aimed at inhibiting normal physiological function.

Infertility and Herd Breeding Problems

Nutritional and other external factors may be involved here, and these must be dealt with if appropriate. As far as the individual animal is concerned, infertility usually requires a constitutional approach. Potentially all the major polychrests may be of use, but some, such as Sepia and Pulsatilla, will feature more prominently in treatments. In dairy herds selective breeding programmes can create the situation where there is a preponderance of particular constitutional types, and in these cases it will be possible to treat a herd problem on the basis of a single constitutional prescription. Previous conventional hormonal treatment in all species may be causing a block to successful treatment and in these cases the use of the same drug in potency will be one way of overcoming this (tautopathy). It should also be noted that the ill effects of these drugs are not confined to the reproductive system, and the use of the potentised form may well also help these wider problems.

The breeding and production requirements of dairy herds can result in a stress on the system that causes a lowering of overall performance which shows itself in longer calving intervals, failure to hold to service, lower milk yields and a higher incidence of all forms of mastitis than would otherwise be encountered. A herd constitutional remedy may be indicated here, but the routine use of Sepia in these circumstances has been shown to have a beneficial effect on all the parameters associated with dairy management. Trial work involving various potencies and time intervals has shown that a single dose of Sepia 200c given 14 days post-partum gave the best results (Williamson).

Abortion, in the absence of specific infections, also calls for a constitutional approach if time allows, although remedies such as Secale Cornutum and Viburnum Opulus will be of use in the more acute situation when the threat of abortion is imminent.

False Pregnancy in the Bitch

The true nature of this condition requires consideration. The carnivore reproductive cycle and system have developed on the basis of a pregnancy following every oestrus, and the condition is only seen when the bitch has not been bred with. To describe not breeding with a bitch as an abuse may seem extreme, but it is certainly an unnatural sequence of events. A false pregnancy could be the body's attempt to return to normal by simulating the normal cycle and allowing a 'safety valve' to operate. It is also worth considering what would be the pack dynamic in the wild, where most females that come into season become pregnant. Those that do not may become involved in the rearing process. Viewed in this way, aggressive conventional treatment of the condition is a form of suppression. Homeopathic remedies are of use in helping the re-adjustment to work through, thereby relieving the clinical condition.

The system of induced ovulation, as seen in felines, allows for the natural cessation of reproductive activity; the condition is therefore not seen in those species, as there is no need for the body to complete a physiological process.

Pregnancy, Parturition and Nursing

Homeopathic support and assistance can be given without risk to the young. There is also the possibility of eugenic treatment of the unborn to remove inherited miasmatic influences. This may be used on a broad basis aimed at the general correction of imbalance, and single consecutive doses of Sulphur, Calc. Carb. and Tuberculinum are given at weekly intervals as soon as pregnancy is confirmed. Sulphur and Tuberculinum are included as agents that cover a broad range of the miasmatic influences, and Calc. Carb. because of its strong psoric connection. Alternatively, the pattern of known specific problems in the dam, for example herpes, can be prevented from being transmitted to the young.

Similarly, treatment of the mother while nursing poses no problems of affecting the young via the milk. Treatment during the later stages of pregnancy will result in an easier birth process, with consequent reduced stress on the mother. Although the causes of mastitis in the farm situation go beyond purely genital considerations, easing of parturition has been shown to have a marked beneficial effect of the subsequent performance of the mother. Although they have not been quantified in other circumstances, these benefits will of course also apply to the non-commercial species.

Major Modalities and Rubrics

The timing, duration and nature of the oestrus are important. The appearance and quantity of any discharges must be noted, as must those of the milk. Mental and behavioural changes associated with hormonal activity are significant, and these will include the attitude of the animal to mating. Reproductive signs and history can give valuable clues when addressing the constitutional or miasmatic aspects of a case.

The repertory has a whole chapter on female genitalia. In addition, some useful rubrics will be found in Mind and Generalities. Rubrics in connection with the mammary glands will be found under Chest.

The human terminology in the repertories refers to 'menses'. While the detailed physiology of the species may vary, the functional aim is the same, and the rubrics may hence be equated with 'oestrus'. There is, of course, no physiological equivalent to the menopause in the domesticated species and here caution must be exercised in using associated rubrics.

Remedies of Major Use

Caulophyllum

Although not considered a major remedy in general terms, it has an important place in the reproductive sphere. It is often used in the last third of pregnancy to help to regulate and facilitate parturition. A 30c dose once weekly is usually employed – care must be exercised over using it more often than that as a pre-emptive treatment, to avoid any proving effect. One of its effects at the time of parturition is to assist the dilation of the cervix and hence it has been used successfully for ringwomb, especially in sheep but also in other species (Cimicifuga may also help in this regard). This effect on the cervix can be utilised to turn a closed pyometra into an open one.

Painful non-productive uterine contractions occur, but there may also be weak contractions, either from exhaustion or linked to a primary inertia. Its discharges are chocolate-coloured. Its failure to act is often indicative of a dead foetus.

There is nervousness and excitability in the picture and animals that will not commence parturition because of this can be helped. It will be helpful in some cases of retained placenta and uterine bleeding.

Its effect on the mammary gland is generally considered to be indirect via easing parturition, but there may be a more direct action and it should be considered in the subclinical mastitis situation.

Sore feet and pain in the small joints are also present in the picture.

Lachesis

A strong keynote of this remedy is < suppressed discharges, and conversely > discharges starting. It thus has a place in the treatment of those conditions associated with chemical contraception, and also in pyometra. It is a left-sided remedy with a marked affinity for the throat, which is sensitive to touch and pressure. Another aspect of the throat is a tendency to vocal expression, which can be marked. There is a dislike of heat, and animals will avoid the sun. All conditions are < sleep.

It is a haemorrhagic remedy and bloody discharges that do not clot are a feature. It is indicated in septic and necrotic states where there is great depression.

Affected tissues are swollen and show a purple-blue tinge. It is a useful remedy in acute mastitis.

Lilium Tigrinum

Its main action is on the urogenital system, and there is a left-sided laterality. Mentally there is a combination of anxiety and bad temper. Animals, especially dogs, are often fat. The animal normally drinks little and often, but the thirst increases before the onset of other symptoms. This is accompanied by the frequent passage of small quantities of urine. There is restlessness, yet there is also an unwillingness to move around. Uterine discharges only appear on movement; they have a strong smell and contain blood, often in clots. This is one of the remedies where a heaviness and dragging downward sensation of the genital organs is reported in humans. It is thus a remedy for uterine prolapse when accompanied by straining. Other uses are in pyometra and infertility, especially when there is inflammation of the left ovary. It is < heat, movement, and consolation and > cold, lying on the left side, and in the open air.

Pulsatilla

This is one of the big constitutional remedies and a major female remedy. Conditions may have a history of beginning at puberty. Pulsatilla animals are friendly with a great desire to please. They love sympathy and fuss, are timid and dislike strange or new situations, and have a low pain threshold. They will often urinate with excitement or fear. Changeability is a keynote on both the mental and physical levels.

Discharges are profuse, bland and white, with possibly a slight yellow-green hue. The thirst is small and is often not increased either by illness or by conventional medications. They generally appear to dislike heat and will actively seek cool places.

There is however some desire for heat, and a factor in their reaction is a dislike of the stuffy atmosphere that often goes with artificial heat. Oestrus can be irregular due to underactivity of the ovaries. False pregnancies are seen frequently in the type, when they will produce large quantities of milk and nurse everything in sight. The type is normally friendly and outgoing but they can become moody during the false pregnancy, with depression and even some signs of aggression. Although they may be upset while pregnant they make good mothers. Mastitis may occur with swelling, heat, tenderness in the glands, and hardness of the teats. Uses include suppressed oestrus, infertility, and nymphomania. It is also indicated in some cases of pyometra, while it has a role in false pregnancy, incontinence, and retained placenta, especially in cattle.

Sepia

This is a predominantly left-sided and female remedy. Its main sphere of action is on the endocrine glands and the uterus. It affects the pituitary-adrenal-gonad triad mentioned above, and tends towards a sexual neutrality. Animals that are neutered at times of high hormonal activity (e.g. pyometra) will often benefit from Sepia.

Mentally they are apathetic and moody and can be bad-tempered. There is a low libido and animals are often passively indifferent to mating.

The whole picture is one of sluggishness, but once they can be stimulated everything improves. False pregnancy where there is depression with little milk production or desire to nurse anything will be helped. They are generally not good mothers and will abandon their offspring. This is again a passive thing with no attempt to kill the young.

Discharges can be of a variable nature but are mainly yellow. There is sensitivity to touch over the pelvic region. Irregular and slight oestrus is seen. The 'bearing down' sensation which is present, together with a general laxity of the tissues, give it indications in abortion and prolapse. Straining may continue after parturition.

Work in cattle has shown that its routine individual use at fourteen days post-partum results in an improved overall reproductive performance. Other clinical indications include pyometra, false pregnancy, infertility, and incontinence in neutered females.

Other Remedies to Consider

Cimicifuga (Actaea Racemosa)
    Irregular, weak and intermittent uterine contractions
    Ovarian inflammation and pain
    Delayed ovulation and reduced discharge during seasons

Phytolacca
    Right-sided
    Mammary glands hard and painful. Abscesses and tumours in glands
    Absence of seasons

Sabina
    Retained placenta
    Bloody, watery uterine discharges
    Post-partum haemorrhage

Urtica Urens
Low potency reduces milk production, high potency increases
Oedema of the mammary glands
Uterine haemorrhage

Ustilago Maydis
Both bright-red and dark uterine discharges. Part clotted
Uterine discharges < movement
Deficient milk production

References

Day, C.E.I. (1985) Control of stillbirths in pigs using homeopathy. *Veterinary Record* **114**(9), 216.

Williamson, A.V. et al. (1995) A trial of Sepia. *British Homeopathic Journal* **84**, 14–20.

Chapter 22

The Male Genital System

General Considerations

This chapter continues the trend of the last two in discussing yet another area of manifestation of sycosis, the miasm which so commonly finds its expression in the urogenital system. Some authorities assert that the sycotic miasm centres around the concept of expansion; as such the genital system plays a pivotal role in its expression, associated as it is with cell division, reproduction, procreation and the increase in size of the social group. One may well ponder on the effect on the organism of removing the organs which are primarily involved in this function; male animals are kept in a state which is less artificial than that of their female counterparts, but it is still an unnatural situation for a male dog never to be given the opportunity of expressing its sexuality. The alternative of surgical neutering may not be a lot worse energetically. Nevertheless it is the authors' advice that castration be viewed critically and avoided wherever possible. Where this is performed for therapeutic reasons such as the control of prostatic hyperplasia or perianal adenomata, the premise applies that this is still not dealing with the underlying imbalance to the vital force; therefore, addressing this by means of homeopathic medicine is not only desirable but probably essential if the sequelae of awakening the deeper levels of disease are to be avoided. In practice, castration is not often identified as a major factor in the development of chronic disease, whereas the same cannot be said of the use of chemical agents to perform the same task, and it is recommended that these agents be used with circumspection.

Hormonal deficiency as a result of castration only seems to clinically affect a minority of individuals – those which by merit of their constitution are most vulnerable. A constitutional prescription may redress this problem; otherwise recourse may be made to organotherapy in the form of low-potency preparations of either male hormones or testis. The sluggishness and poor hair coat which afflicts these patients may be considerably relieved thereby.

The suppression of sexuality which mankind imposes on domestic pets may be reflected in an awakening of the cancer miasm, with testicular and prostatic cancer the inevitable sequelae. It is a matter for debate whether surgery will spare the animal the greater effects of this suppression or not.

If Psora is responsible for deficiency, then entire males with no libido may be considered to be under the influence of this miasm; conversely, Sycosis may be expected to be reflected in an increased libido. However, an increased sex drive is just as commonly part of a Tubercular picture and indeed the more commonly used remedies for this problem tend to be Tubercular. In the wild, it is normal for a sexually mature male to have free range to seek out potential mates. The restriction inherent in the keeping of domestic pets redirects this energy into the over-sexual states expressed in the tubercular miasm. The syphilitic miasm is responsible for the retention of testes in developing animals, and while it is difficult to be completely objective in this situation, it is the authors' opinion that treatment of animals so affected with anti-syphilitic homeopathic medicines such as Aurum Metallicum and Clematis Erecta is frequently effective in encouraging normal positioning of the testes. There is of course an ethical issue surrounding this area due to the hereditary nature of such developmental abnormalities. In theory, homeopathic treatment of the underlying miasmatic tendency should ensure that this genetic propensity is not transferred to offspring although there is as yet no evidence for or against this premise, and the issue remains one of personal choice by the veterinary surgeon.

Major Modalities and Rubrics

The prostate gland is afforded its own chapter in the repertory, whereas the rest of the male genital system is represented under 'Male genitalia/sex'. Swelling and inflammation of the respective organs may be used as symptoms for analysis, as well as the contrary states of atrophy and induration. In the case of the testes, laterality is significant and retention of testes is represented by the rubric 'retraction', though 'cryptorchidism' is also available in newer repertories. Discharges from prepuce are noted with their colour and consistency, although discharges from the urethra are found in the specific section accorded to it. Modalities and lesions such as condylomata or ulcers are represented in sections relating to the relevant organs. Libido is described as 'sexual desire' and rubrics covering masturbation can be useful. Phimosis and paraphimosis can be found under that heading in the repertory.

Where there is prostatic enlargement the effect on urination or defaecation can be a significant factor in making a homeopathic prescription, though caution should be exerted in extrapolating human symptomatology, given the slightly different anatomy in the respective species.

Remedies of Major Use

Pulsatilla

Although typically regarded as a 'female' remedy, Pulsatilla has many symptoms associated with the male genital system. Perhaps most important are the symptoms of prostatitis, particularly the acute form. The thick, bland, mucopurulent discharges of Pulsatilla find expression through the urethra, and there is pain on urination. The discharge may also be bloody, and prostatitis may be accompanied by arthritic pain in the right hip. Orchitis is also a part of the Pulsatilla picture, especially if it is right-sided.

Thuja

This major anti-sycotic medicine finds use in virtually any problem associated with the male genital system; balanoposthitis with profuse yellow or green discharge, prostatic enlargement and chronic induration of the testes are all represented in its materia medica. Thuja is indicated in benign tumours and condylomata, so warts or equine sarcoids on and around the prepuce and benign tumours of the testes may be indications for its use.

Mercurius Solubilis

The purulent inflammations and ulcerations characteristic of Mercury are exhibited in the male genital system as, in particular, a purulent balanoposthitis, with ulcerative lesions on penis or prepuce, and a greenish or yellow mucopurulent discharge, often with blood; the ulcers too will bleed if handled. The pain associated with this may be a factor in the phimosis or paraphimosis for which this remedy is indicated. There is great swelling of the prepuce and there may be painful orchitis.

Conium Maculatum

In humans, Conium is indicated in old men where the sexual desire has been repressed, either as a result of absence or of loss of a sexual

233

partner. Because entire male animals, particularly dogs, may be considered to undergo a similar experience, in later life Conium is frequently indicated. Prostatic enlargement causes interference with the passage of urine, which is intermittent; urine flows, stops and then flows again; there may also be dribbling of urine. Conium is associated with enlargement and subsequent atrophy and induration of the testes, also with cancerous affections generally. It is therefore of prime consideration in cancer of the testes or prostate. There is concomitant weakness of the hind legs and despite the age of the patients sexual desire may still be high, though the ability is lacking.

Tarentula Hispanica

This spider remedy is a major antituberculinic, and it exhibits the hyperactivity characteristic of this miasm. However, it finds its expression particularly in the sexual sphere. There is increased libido, the affected animal mounting people, other animals and inanimate objects and masturbating openly. The genitals are sensitive, and perhaps as a consequence of the persistent sexual excitement there may be prostatitis. The oversexed adolescent dog who is exuberant and destructive will frequently respond to this remedy. Tarentula has an interesting sensitivity to colours and may take an aversion to a particular item of clothing worn by an owner; red and green are commonly the colours involved, and the wearer may well find herself being mounted by the Tarentula dog. There is also a sensitivity to music, and a calming effect may be noted in the Tarentula patient, particularly by music with a consistent rhythm.

Other Remedies to Consider

Agnus Castus
    Impotence, loss of sexual desire
    Premature old age as a result of overuse sexually
    Testes cold, small flaccid

Clematis Erecta
    Orchitis, especially right testis
    Retained testes
    Dribbling after urination

Lycopodium
   Enlarged prostate, prostatitis
   Impotence; premature ejaculation
   Increased libido

Rhododendron
   Orchitis; testes swollen, painful
   Induration of testes
   Pain in testes > motion, < before storm or change in weather

Sabal Serrulata
   Senile hyperplasia of prostate
   Cystitis from prostatic hypertrophy
   Epididymitis

Chapter 23

The Musculoskeletal System

General Considerations

This anatomical classification covers muscles, bones, joints and their associated nervous supply; however, as paralysis is included in Chapter 23, on the nervous system, the present discussion will exclude this symptom.

Osteoarthrosis and other similar conditions represent one of the most common reasons for animal owners to consult a homeopathic veterinary surgeon; firstly because it is a field in which homeopathy can be very effective, and secondly because the harmful side effects of the non-steroidal inflammatory drugs (NSAIDs) and of corticosteroids themselves are well documented and well known by the public at large. Add to this the fact that most of the patients who develop these diseases are of advancing years and the importance of using a therapy which does no harm becomes increasingly apparent. As far as NSAIDs are concerned, sadly these drugs do seem to antidote homeopathy quite seriously. It is therefore necessary to remove these medicines from the therapeutic regime before the effect of homeopathic remedies can be expected to reach their full potential. Less antidotal seems to be aspirin, and in dogs this medicine may be used as a stepping stone to relying on homeopathy alone. In horses and dogs, chondroprotective agents such as glucosamine or chondroitin sulphate do not seem to be antidotal, nor does therapy using agents such as magnetic collars or bandages.

Joint disease is generally regarded as a manifestation of Sycosis and in the main this generalisation holds true, especially where there is overproduction causing swelling of the joints or exostosis. However, lack of joint fluid may be considered as a deficiency state and therefore psoric, and destructive lesions such as osteochondritis dissecans (OCD) are without doubt manifestations of Syphilis.

It might however be pertinent at this point to enlarge on the effect of diet on the canine locomotor system. It is considered by some, the authors among them, that the rearing of puppies on commercial diets results in young animals who grow too quickly, with inadequate

236

nutrient availability to support this. The consequence is that bone and cartilage are of poor quality and ligaments are lax. Loose intervertebral ligaments cause fixations of the facet joints, which in turn lead to irritation of the roots of the nerves supplying muscles in specific areas. The resulting tension in the associated muscles causes excess pressure to be exerted on the joint around which they function, often in an asymmetric direction. In the case of the hip joint, this mechanism is what causes the pectineus muscle to contract; the result is excess pressure on a joint which is not structurally sound enough to cope with it. Add to this the effects of genetically poor conformation and excess weight bearing, and hip dysplasia results; a similar process in the forelegs results in the development of such conditions as OCD of the elbow joint and fragmentation of the coronoid process.

In the treatment of such conditions, therefore, it is highly advantageous to add chiropractic manipulation to the regime of treatment. Similarly, chronic strains of the long head of the triceps can only be fully resolved if the associated fixations of the cervico-thoracic spine are released. In horses, similar mechanisms may be involved in the pathogenesis of many chronic lamenesses. Attention to correct shoeing and saddling can be essential if resolution of the problems is to be achieved. In the UK, the McTimoney animal chiropractors, who train for three years as human chiropractors before undergoing a further two years instruction in animal manipulation, may be relied on to adequately address these issues. It will be seen from the foregoing that the musculoskeletal system should be viewed as a finely balanced dynamic system comprising the limbs and spine; bones, ligaments and muscular tissues. Homeopathic treatment may sometimes therefore be just one therapy in a multidisciplinary approach to such problems.

As a nutritional footnote, the authors also consider that dogs and cats need an exogenous source of vitamin C, and the mechanics of the degenerative processes described above are exacerbated by the low levels of vitamin C in most commercial diets. If owners cannot be persuaded to feed the raw vegetables and fruit which comprise part of the 'BARF' diet, then supplementation is to be recommended.

Major Modalities and Rubrics

It is not always possible to elucidate whether an animal is suffering from pain; however, where this is clear, the rubrics 'Extremities; pain' and its sub-rubrics are of value. Otherwise the rubrics of 'Stiffness' must be reverted to, although these appear to be less appropriate when dealing with animals than with their human counterparts. Modalities appertaining to movement are critical, particularly aggravation or amelioration from first movement or continued movement; similarly, the effect of rest and in particular rest after exercise. Weather modalities also are important; the effect of cold damp weather, warm dry weather, cold dry weather, windy weather and the effect of a change of weather are all significant. Symptoms may be modulated by local warmth or cold applications.

Pathology of the area affected includes swelling and deformity of joints, and exostoses.

Laterality of limb involvement may be specific for certain remedies, and diagonal patterns of lameness are significant. Ledum, for instance, has pain in the left shoulder accompanied by pain in the right hip.

Locality of pain or pathology is also important, some remedies having a predilection for a particular joint or a specific area of the spine. Actea Spicata, for instance, has a predilection for the carpal joint, whereas Tellurium has pain in the spine from the last cervical to the fifth dorsal vertebra.

When extrapolating from human material, there is some confusion as to whether 'forefeet' equates with 'hands'. It is the authors' contention that this approximation often does hold true, but flexibility in interpretation is advised if valuable rubrics are not to be missed. Sometimes the use of 'foot' for 'forefeet' is justified, at other times it is not. Of significance is the question as to whether the symptoms are consequent of weight bearing or not. If the involvement of the forefeet alone cannot easily be explained then it is admissible to look at the rubrics for 'hand'. If it is just part of a general arthritic condition affecting all weight-bearing joints then it is safer to confine the repertorisation to rubrics for the feet.

While weakness of limbs is certainly a symptom which is relevant to the musculoskeletal system, and rubrics under 'Extremities; weakness' are useful, it is more fully discussed under the nervous system in Chapter 24.

Remedies of Major Use

Pulsatilla

The locomotor symptoms of Pulsatilla reflect its changeability in producing a wandering lameness, pains moving from joint to joint and limb to limb. Symptoms are aggravated by damp weather and also in hot weather. Gentle movement in the open air ameliorates symptoms, and cool applications ameliorate. There is a predilection for the right hip or stifle but pains are worse lying on the left or painless side; there is also pain at the lumbosacral junction.

Calcarea Carbonica

Joint affections in Calc. Carb. show pain which is aggravated by cold damp weather and by getting wet. There is pain and swelling of affected joints, especially the stifles, and exostoses are a prominent feature. Exostoses in the form of spondylosis are associated with pain and stiffness of the cervical and lumbar spine in particular. Pain and stiffness generally are relieved by motion and lying on the painful side.

The chilliness of Calc. Carb. is reflected in the feet, which feel cold and damp.

Causticum

Causticum shows deformity of the joints and pain, and stiffness which is only partially relieved by motion. Arthritic changes in the spine result in weakness of the hind legs, sometimes with associated urinary or faecal incontinence. Many aged dogs exhibit this picture and it is in that age group where Causticum finds its most common usage. The weather modalities of Causticum may be confusing; according to most homeopathic text books, there is aggravation in cold dry weather and amelioration in damp weather. However, it may present in the opposite way and it is the authors' experience that Causticum is most commonly indicated where there is amelioration in cold dry weather. However, the dog which chooses to lie on damp grass may also require this remedy. Mentally, Causticum may exhibit irritability, but the characteristic protectiveness to the family and sympathetic nature are more prominent features. Warts on the face are another keynote to this remedy.

Rhus Toxicodendron

After Arnica, Rhus Tox. is perhaps the most commonly prescribed homeopathic medicine, due to its reputation in the treatment of arthritis. Joint pain and back pain are major features and the modalities are distinctive; pains are worse on first movement but better for continued movement. However, as fatigue sets in the pain and stiffness returns. The aggravation from rest which characterises Rhus Tox. leads to the description 'worse after rest after exercise'. The other strong guiding modality to Rhus Tox. is its aggravation in cold and damp weather; it is also worse for getting wet, and like Pulsatilla will often try and prevent getting its feet wet by avoiding walking through puddles. Wherever these movement and weather modalities are clear, Rhus Tox. will bring relief, whether the problem involves muscles, tendons, ligaments or fasciae.

There is also aggravation before thunderstorms; indeed there may be fear of thunder.

Night-time aggravation, coupled with the effect of rest, means that night is the worst time for the Rhus Tox. patient; in an effort to get comfortable the animal changes position frequently, or gets up and walks round to ease the discomfort. Initially this is effective, but as soon as the patient lies down again the pain returns and another cycle of rest and movement begins. The result of this is an animal which exhibits nocturnal restlessness, the animal intermittently pacing around and frequently changing its resting place. Perhaps not surprisingly the Rhus Tox. patient at this stage is somewhat irritable, but even so the innate good humour of this remedy will shine through. On the general level, Rhus Tox. is chilly, thirsty and craves milk.

Used at low potency at a local level, Rhus Tox. can be highly efficacious in these situations. However, it should be noted that these movement and weather modalities are shared by other homeopathic medicines, so for long-lasting cures, as opposed to palliation, prescription on a more constitutional level will be required. Nevertheless, even used on a local basis, Rhus Tox. can be of immense value in the treatment of joint pain in animals, and its reputation in this field is well justified.

Bryonia Alba

Bryonia is sometimes considered to be the opposite of Rhus Tox. and indeed its modalities are contrary to Rhus. Firstly, Bryonia is worse for any movement; in the more severe cases there is reluctance to move at all and in less severe cases the further the animal walks the more lame it becomes. Secondly, Bryonia pains are worse for warmth and ameliorated in wet weather, though cold dry weather may also aggravate. As the essence of Bryonia is dryness, it may be the dryness which is the important factor in these weather modalities. There is also a peculiar amelioration by firm pressure, so that the Bryonia patient tends to lie with the affected limb underneath it. In such a state of discomfort, it is not surprising that Bryonia is irritable and averse to being disturbed. Patients are often described as being 'rigid of fibre', and there is a characteristic thirst for large quantities at long intervals.

Bryonia is often needed after Rhus Tox. and this is because the latter is sometimes observed to undergo what is known as a reversal of modalities. The patient who has responded to Rhus Tox. thus begins to show modalities more akin to Bryonia, and switching the prescription to Bryonia takes the case further on along the path of improvement. Reversal may then occur again, with the result that over a period of time the two remedies are alternated, all the time with a steady improvement in the patient.

Other Remedies to Consider

Arnica Montana
> Stiffness and pain in back and limbs 'as if bruised'
> Restless in bed, as cannot get comfortable
> < Cold and damp weather, exertion

Calcarea Fluorica
> Exostoses; 'splints' and ringbone in horses
> Chronic synovitis of the stifle; old cruciate ligament injuries
> < cold and damp weather, change of weather. Generally worse for heat

Caulophyllum
> Arthritis of small joints, especially phalanges
> Joint pains after parturition
> Postparturient swellings of fetlocks in cattle

Conium Maculatum
> Pain between shoulders
> Aching in lumbar and sacral region
> Coccydinia (pain in tail)

Ledum Palustre
> Sprains of hocks
> Pains > cold applications but patient generally chilly
> Arthritis begins in hind feet and travels upwards

Ruta Graveolens
> Bursitis, tendinitis
> Contractions of toes
> Arthritic pains, especially due to overuse, chronic sprains
> < cold and damp weather, exertion

Chapter 24

The Nervous System

General Considerations

The nervous system is, in many ways, the most susceptible of all to the effects of upsets in other systems, as well as to more direct effects. Thus toxaemia arising from liver or kidney disease will produce symptoms, and damage to nerves is almost inevitable in any major trauma incident. If the spinal column is involved, the production of oedema due to injury can aggravate nerve damage due to the pressure created, and Apis is a valuable remedy in these circumstances. But there is an involvement in the chronic disease picture as well. The system has a strong connection with the psoric miasm. Due to the embryological development of the central nervous system from the primordial skin tissue there is a tendency for suppression of psora to show as a nervous disorder. Due to the intrinsic nature of psora (Chapter 11) manifesting as a failure or reduction of function, this will result in paralysis or muscular weakness. Some cases of Bell's palsy and Horner's syndrome will arise in this way. Conversely, successful treatment of nervous conditions may result in the appearance of skin symptoms. The other suppressive connection of the system involves the syphilitic miasm: one of the structures that will be attacked as a result of the blocking of an outlet for the syphilitic miasm is the meninges, and this results in the destructive effects associated with the miasm involving the nervous system.

Epilepsy

It is important to differentiate between epilepsy and convulsions from some other cause. True idiopathic epilepsy is essentially part of a chronic condition and its treatment should be approached from the constitutional angle. The 'seesaw' pattern found in other circumstances between the lungs and the skin also occurs here between the nervous system and the skin. Conventionally, a definite hereditary connection is recognised in many conditions, of which epilepsy is one. But it must be remembered that in homeopathic terms it is possible for there to be the passage of miasmatic influences through the generations which is not hereditary in the sense of dominant and recessive genes etc., although nonetheless real for all that. It is these animals that will most easily become clinical cases following some trigger or suppressive treatment. Vaccination is one major agent here, especially if that has produced signs in other systems that have been suppressed. Aetiological considerations in general are particularly valuable in the approach to epilepsy.

One of the major problems in the treatment of epilepsy is that, due to the dramatic and distressing nature of the symptom, there is often great reluctance on the part of both veterinary surgeon and owner to lighten any control of the convulsions that has been established. While this is understandable, it must be realised that such control is a form of suppression in the homeopathic sense, and will hence militate against a successful cure of the condition.

Stroke and 'Stroke Syndrome'

Although genuine strokes do occur in animals, in many cases this is not the same syndrome as occurs in humans, and should more accurately be described as 'vestibular syndrome'. It is primarily a condition of the older animal. In homeopathic terms it is an acute disease. There is no primary nervous lesion, and it would appear to be a case of the nervous function being influenced by primary malfunction in another system. The cardiovascular system is the most likely although the exact mechanism is unclear, and there appears to be a lipaemia associated with some cases. The effect on the nervous system involves the vestibular apparatus. Initial treatment is with remedies such as Aconite, Arnica and Belladona. Cerebral anoxia results in oedema, and as above, Apis should be considered. Subsequent therapy is based on the presenting picture.

Chronic Degenerative Radiculomyelopathy (CDRM)

Now being called merely 'degenerative myelopathy' in some quarters, there is evidence to suggest that repeated booster vaccination may have a role in the aetiology of this syndrome (CHC Survey). It is primarily a syphilitic/psoric condition. In addition to remedies selected on the presenting picture, such as Conium and Lathyrus, the miasmatic nosodes have a role in treatment. As the condition involves destruction of the myelin sheath, the use of Syphilinum to halt the process can be particularly helpful. Of equal importance is supplementation with vitamins C and E. It is one of the conditions in which a combination of homeopathy and acupuncture may yield the best results, with the latter therapy being used to give a local stimulation to the spinal nerves.

Neoplasia

The first consideration involves the location of the growth, which governs the approach to treatment. Primary neoplasia does arise within the nervous tissue, but the system can be severely affected by pressure from pathology in other tissues. In both cases the miasmatic implications must be addressed (Chapter 30), as the miasmatic imbalances (Chapter 11) are crucial to the development of neoplasia. However, the need to deal with pathology in the first case, as against the effects of damage and pressure on the nerves in the latter, will lead to different support remedies being indicated in each situation.

Major Modalities and Rubrics

Signs and symptoms include:

- loss or perversion of muscular function
- loss of consciousness
- convulsions
- hypo- and hyper-aesthesia
- behavioural changes
- loss of senses
- postural abnormalities

In the repertory, rubrics of relevance to the above will be found in all sections. The chapter on vertigo contains some rubrics that can be useful in animals, but in the main the required rubrics will be found in the chapters relating to the systems in which the signs are manifest. Movement is an important modality. Any tendency to fall, or a tilting of the head, may display laterality. In veterinary medicine many of the pain rubrics are unusable but the modalities of touch and heat in relation to pain are the most significant. Behavioural changes may occur as a result of changes in the senses. A large section on convulsions will be found in the Generals chapter, although references will also be found in other places, for example 'Respiration; difficult; convulsions, during'.

244

In cases of epilepsy the exact features of the convulsions must be investigated, including any sexual connections in relation to coition or thwarted sexual desire. Phases of the moon can also influence the timing of convulsions, and the relevant rubrics will also be found in the Generals chapter.

Remedies of Major Use

Belladonna

The action here is on the central nervous system. Nervous signs associated with hyperthermia are common, and its use in heatstroke and high fevers is beneficial. Signs are accompanied by an accelerated, bounding pulse and great heat. On occasion the beat of the heart can be easily seen on the thoracic wall. Conditions are of sudden onset, and it has a use in cerebral haemorrhage and the canine stroke syndrome.

Convulsions of all types may be helped, from true epilepsy to hypo-calcaemia and hypomagnesaemia. (Milk fever and staggers will still need mineral replacement, as will eclampsia in the bitch.) Epileptic attacks are often preceded by restlessness. There is aggression, twitching of muscles around the head, and falling. Animals in convulsions are often vocal, with screaming and bellowing.

Cuprum Metallicum

The action on the nerves is based around the cerebrospinal axis. The effect is to produce spasms and cramps. There is much twitching of the muscles and whole groups can be seen in spasm. When the animal is asleep this causes jerking of the limbs. Convulsions also occur, beginning in the legs and moving up to the body.

There is great spasm of the muscles, the jaws become locked, and much saliva is produced. There is a tendency to fall forwards, and during convulsions the head is turned to one side, although there is no marked preference as to which. Howling or bellowing are often heard. After fits there is great prostration.

This is a remedy that shows a strong relationship between the skin and the CNS.

Suppression of skin eruptions and normal discharges can trigger fits. Convulsions as a result of any incident causing anoxia to the medulla may respond.

All conditions are sudden in onset and tend to be violent. Hyper-sensitivity is a general feature. Another general feature of Cuprum Met.

245

is that any other medication given to the patient will cause a reaction, although this is not necessarily curative.

Gelsemium

The affinity with the nervous system is evident on both the mental and physical levels. It figures in rubrics concerned with aetiologies involving both fear and excitement, and unless corrected often leads to physical changes. There is motor weakness that progresses to paralysis, and the weakness is accompanied by trembling of the affected muscles. Pedal reflexes are reduced and there is an unsteady and uncoordinated movement. Incontinence of faeces and/or urine can accompany the more generalised weakness seen in the hind limbs. Paralysis of single parts can occur and the eyelids will appear slack, while nystagmus may be seen. Painful swellings of the joints can occur, especially of the stifle. In generalised conditions there is great depression and lassitude with aching in all muscles, but particularly in the shoulders. It is a thirstless remedy.

Hypericum

This is the most commonly used and successful remedy for damage to nerves. Although its main sphere of action is on the peripheral nerves, it is also effective in cases of damage to the central nervous system. The meninges are also affected. There is a general picture of pain and sensitivity rather than paralysis, the lower end of the spine being particularly affected. The pain is < movement, and affected parts tend towards spasm. Postoperative pain can be controlled by it. A major use is in conjunction with Arnica in cases of injury and Ledum where there are puncture wounds. This latter is of use in cases of actual or threatened tetanus. As a local application it is often mixed with Calendula. This combination assists in reducing the tendency of an animal to self-mutilate a sore while stimulating the healing of the tissues.

Plumbum Metallicum

There is an action here on both the spinal cord and the peripheral parts. A marked feature is paralysis of single parts, and it has given good results in radial paralysis.

Although there is a special affinity with the front limbs in relation to paralysis, CDRM may also benefit, as muscle atrophy is seen as well as loss of nerve function.

Conditions are often of slow onset, and the gradual onset of loco-motor ataxia is seen.

In its action on the central nerves it produces convulsions which are preceded by vertigo. Following convulsions there is mental depression and deep sleeping which in an extreme case may progress to coma. There is a marked turning of the head to the right after a fit. Nervous symptoms due to neoplasia of the CNS are an indication.

Initially conditions may show pain and hyperaesthesia before progressing to paralysis.

Other Remedies to Consider

Bufo
   Tendency towards aggression develops
   Convulsions < night and sleep. Aggression before convulsions
   Cramping of muscles
   Hypersexuality

Cicuta Virosa
   Upsets of balance
   Head and neck twisted backwards during convulsions
   Twitching and spasms of muscles
   Pupils contract and dilate alternately

Conium
   Ascending paralysis
   Weakness of limbs, especially the hind
   Trembling of fore limbs
   Aetiology of bruising to spinal cord and associated nerves
   Obturator (calving) paralysis in cattle

Hyoscyamus
   Head shaking in horses
   Dilated pupils
   Obscene behaviour (spraying in cats)
   Muscular spasms during convulsions. Facial twitching

Lathyrus
   Unsteady gait. Loss of spatial awareness
   Atrophy of muscle groups
   Increased but incoordinated reflexes

Opium
  Depressed nervous responses
  Contracted pupils
  Painless and paralysis

Stramonium
  Rhythmic movement of limbs
  Upset by bright lights
  Staggering gait and falling forward

References

Canine Health Concern Survey, 1997.
Holcombe, A.W. (1982) *Spasms and Convulsions. An Abridged Repertory.* New Delhi: World Homeopathic Links.

Chapter 25

The Cardiovascular System

General Considerations

Although vascular disease is increasingly recognised in domestic animals, it is the heart which is most frequently involved in diseases of this body system, and which will therefore be mainly considered in this chapter. Classically, cardiac problems are considered to be part of the sycotic miasm and this is borne out by the preponderance of vegetative lesions in cardiac pathology. With the growing evidence for an immune-mediated basis for much of cardiac pathology, and the suggested link between vaccination and immune disorders, the sycotic influence becomes clearer. It nevertheless has to be said that degenerative disease such as cardiomyopathy would lead one to consider Syphilis as the major miasm involved, and autoimmune disease generally is often considered to be syphilitic. As a deficiency state, simple heart weakness may be considered to be psoric. In terms of diet, the provision of fresh raw foods may be beneficial; as previously discussed, many commercial diets contain measurable amounts of salt and perpetuating a dietary imbalance will constitute an obstacle to cure.

By the time disease has reached this most fundamental of levels, it may be inferred that the vital force has been severely weakened and therefore not able to respond fully to higher potencies. Perhaps this is why much homeopathic medicine in this field concentrates on local prescriptions of low potency preparations or mother tinctures. Similarly, the organism may not be able to respond on a constitutional level alone. The authors' management of these cases generally involves using both levels of prescribing and this is often very successful, although reliance on the low potency preparations seems to be the norm towards the end of a patient's life.

This is an area where conventional therapy rarely seems to antidote homeopathy, one possible exception being material doses of digitalis and its analogues. Diuretics and ACE inhibitors do not appear to interfere with the action of the homeopathic medicines, and this is therefore an area where the two forms of therapy may be considered complementary. Nevertheless, it is usually possible to reduce and eventually stop conventional medication after homeopathic therapy begins to take effect. If some form of diuretic is still required, then herbal dandelion tablets can provide a viable alternative to frusemide. An added advantage of this is that, in contrast to the latter, dandelion contains significant levels of potassium and does not therefore induce hypokalaemia.

As for dosage regimes of low potency preparations, normal homeopathic rules apply; however, with mother tinctures there does seem to be a dose-related response, so doses may need to take into account the bodyweight of the patient. Again, while there is considerable variation in individual response to homeopathy, it is often possible to dose even old dogs only intermittently; 10 days of treatment at the beginning of each month is a pattern used with success by the authors. One might expect that complete cure would not be possible using low potency preparations, and certainly palliation is often the best that one can expect in cardiac patients. However, the power of the low potencies and mother tinctures should not be underestimated. One of the authors (P.G.) has seen complete atrioventricular block in a cat completely resolved by one dose of a mother tincture. It does not therefore follow that all patients have to remain on medication, orthodox or homeopathic, permanently.

Major Modalities and Rubrics

Assessment of the cardiovascular system for homeopathic prescribing parallels that for orthodox prescribing, and such techniques as electrocardiography, radiography and ultrasonography should be no less a part of the assessment than with a conventional approach. Valuable information may be obtained thus, not only in terms of making a diagnosis, but also as a way of increasing the accuracy of the homeopathic prescription. By adding to the amount of information available to the prescriber, the repertory may be used more precisely. Similarly, all the information one would collect for a full clinical assessment is also required for the homeopathic treatment of a cardiac condition – size and shape of the heart, auscultation of murmurs and arrhythmias, detection of fluid build-up in the thorax, abdomen or other areas, and character and rate of pulse and respiration. However, the observation of modalities in the assessment of these parameters bears the same importance as with any other symptom in a homeopathic assessment. It is worth noting that most heart medicines show aggravation by warmth and by exertion.

Historically, the heart does not have its own section of the repertory, rubrics relevant to cardiovascular disease being found primarily under the headings of 'Chest' and 'Generalities'. However, other symptoms are dotted around the relevant sections, such as 'Abdomen; dropsy' (under which is the sub-rubric of 'Ascites').

The Chest section contains several rubrics appertaining to pathology such as dilatation of the heart, fatty degeneration, arteriosclerosis of coronary arteries and murmurs, also 'Heart; complaints of' and 'Heart failure'. Symptoms of cardiovascular disease are covered by pain, angina, dropsy and edema (sic). Pulse rate, rhythm and character are dealt with under 'Generalities', although one interesting rubric of 'Ceases; as if heart would cease' is included under the Chest, and another, of 'Mind; delusions; heart; stops beating when sitting' appears in the Mind section. Finally, the sections of 'Cough' and 'Respiration' yield valuable rubrics.

It should be noted that Murphy's repertory includes a separate chapter for the heart.

Remedies of Major Use

Ammonium Carbonicum

Animals requiring Ammon. Carb. are usually fat middle-aged or old patients and they are weak and sluggish. Patients also have wheezing respirations and great difficulty in breathing, exacerbated by the slightest effort. Warm rooms aggravate the symptoms and cool air ameliorates them. However, generally Ammon. Carb. is chilly, so seeks the warmth. There is a dry or wheezing cough which is worse at 3-4 a.m. and on cold damp, particularly cloudy, days. The cough may also be rattly. Auscultation reveals a weak heart and correspondingly the pulse is weak. There is palpitation from the slightest exertion. Pulmonary oedema and emphysema may also be present. Concomitant symptoms may include chronic upper respiratory disease with obstruction of the nostrils, especially at night, and urinary incontinence.

Spongia Tosta

Spongia is one of the most important homeopathic medicines where the overriding symptom is that of a cardiac cough. The cough of Spongia is variously described as 'hollow', 'barking' or 'sawing', indeed one particularly imaginative, though also very accurate, description is that of the sound of a saw going through wood. The cough is worse for excitement; as soon as the dog gets excited in any way, it starts coughing. Breathing is also difficult and the patient may wake at night with a feeling of suffocation. Not surprisingly the mental state with this remedy is one of fear and anxiety. Symptoms are worse for sitting up and relieved by lying down, so the affected animal may choose to lie on its chest rather than sit up. The cough is relieved by drinking water and some dogs do seem to learn this, heading straight for the water bowl when the cough begins. Similarly the cough may be ameliorated by eating. Cardiac disease leading to these symptoms may include valvular lesions or hypertrophy, and the pulse is variably described as full or feeble. However, it is the characteristic cough with its specific modalities which will lead to the successful employment of this remedy.

Cactus Grandiflora

This is another remedy for cardiac coughs, but with Cactus the cough is far less severe. It is the irritating dry cough which the patient in the early stages of cardiac insufficiency will exhibit. The cough is worse at night and quite often will disappear completely during the daytime, though there is also a characteristic worsening at 11 a.m. which has been found to be useful in prescribing this remedy. Cactus is also one of the major remedies in humans for angina pectoris, where the pain is described as being like an iron band around the chest. A symptom picture which corresponds to this is occasionally observed in dogs in particular, where the patient screams and raises its left foreleg. This may reflect the referred pain in the left arm reported by humans, and certainly such episodes can be eliminated by treatment with Cactus in homeopathic potency. Latrodectus has similar symptoms. Once again the pathology which leads to symptoms requiring Cactus is not specific, though valvular lesions, particularly of the mitral valve, are common and the pulse is generally weak and intermittent.

Crataegus Oxyacantha

This is without doubt the most commonly used 'cardiac' medicine in the homeopathic materia medica. As a mother tincture or low potency preparation it has a fairly non-specific tonic effect on the heart, and this is apparent when one reads any description of the medicine in a standard homeopathic materia medica. There may be valvular murmurs, dilatation of the heart, fluid retention, cough and arteriosclerosis; as far as the latter is concerned, Crataegus has a reputation for dissolving arteriosclerotic deposits in humans. However, like all homeopathic medicines, there are symptoms individual to Crataegus, notably extreme dyspnoea on the slightest exertion but without much increase in pulse rate. The pulse itself may be rapid, irregular, weak and intermittent. Symptoms are better in fresh air and for rest. Mentally the patient is often irritable and bad-tempered. Crataegus then may be used as a general 'heart tonic' and may be extremely useful in those elderly patients who just require a little cardiac support and where there are not enough specific symptoms to suggest another remedy.

Adonis Vernalis

The keynote to Adonis is fluid retention. Where the major presenting symptom is of ascites, oedema or hydrothorax, Adonis in tincture or low potency can be extremely effective. As with many cardiac medicines, there may be unsteadiness on rising, dyspnoea and weakness, and the heart may be affected by myocarditis, cardiomyopathy or particularly valvular disease, but if the predominating effect of any of these is fluid retention, then Adonis is indicated. Pulse is rapid and irregular, but paradoxically the symptoms of Adonis are better for exertion and worse for cold.

Other Remedies to Consider

Baryta Muriatica
Syncope
Arteriosclerosis, aneurysm
Senility

Convallaria Majalis
Irregularities of rhythm
Cardiac dilatation
Heart ceases beating, then starts suddenly again

Digitalis Purpurea
Pulse slow, weak, intermittent
Least movement causes palpitation
Use in potency, e.g. 30c

Laurocerasus
   Cyanosis
   Tickling cough < lying down, at night
   Mitral regurgitation

Naja Trepudians
   Cough < after lying down
   Cardiac damage after infectious disease, valvular lesions
   Pulse slow, irregular

Chapter 26

The Endocrine System

General Considerations

The endocrine system is the system most closely linked to the homeostatic functions of the body. Because of this there are inevitably close functional links to other systems, such as the immune system, and assaults on those systems can lead, in addition to other consequences, to upsets of endocrine function. This central role in the maintenance of what Hahnemann described as the 'unimpeded progress of life' implies a high degree of control in the functioning of the system. The basic influence behind the function is, of course, the vital force, and the endocrine system is one of the primary pathways through which the force is manifest. Weakness and failure of function are now considered to be the characteristics of the psoric miasm, and many clinical conditions arise as a result of the failures of function induced by its action. Failures of the orchestration and control of the systems necessary for the maintenance of homeostasis are closely linked to the essence of the psoric miasm, and thus in cases of chronic disease involving the endocrine system it is often found that the influence of the psoric miasm is a major factor.

Another consequence of the central role of the system in the maintenance of functional normality is that when the balance of the system is disturbed, the effects are often widespread through the body. Thus many of the polychrests will be found to be of major use in the treatment of such conditions.

Apart from the challenges to the system as a result of recognised disease agents, there are certain procedures of a routine nature that can have profound effects on the system. The first of these is vaccination. Although in this instance the basic assault is on the immune system, nevertheless the endocrine system is involved via an effect primarily on the thyroid gland. This will in many cases create a hypothyroid state, although a hyperfunctional condition can often arise. As discussed in Chapter 21, neutering of either sex has an effect on the pituitary, the effect being potentially greater the more mature the animal is at the time of the interference. In all cases where there is an aetiology involving suppression of sexual function by any means, the mechanism of an effect as a result of an upset to the pituitary function should be considered. It makes no difference whether the suppression is surgical or chemical. In other situations, primarily those linked to food production, man's priorities will result in artificial stimulation or adjustment of the sexual cycle. While these activities may be regarded as more 'natural', since they accord with nature's broad aims of reproduction, problems can still arise as a result of these interventions, as the use of chemical agents to regulate oestrus can still be a suppressive procedure.

The endocrine system has given the materia medica a number of important remedies derived from the healthy tissues of various glands (sarcodes). Although all have their own remedy pictures, one of their uses is as a means of regulating glandular function. In this particular context the definition of high and low potency is different to that which is generally employed (Chapter 8). In relation to the use of sarcodes the point of differentiation is found at 7c, and the action of the sarcode varies on either side of that. It is found that low potencies (below 7c) can have the effect of stimulating glandular function while high potencies (above 7c) produce an inhibitory effect in proportion to the potency. Standard preparations are commonly used across all species but it has been suggested that species-specific remedies may have a greater effect (Elliott 1995), and this may also hold true for their use as remedies generally. Various hormonal preparations are used in conventional medicine for both hormonal and non-hormonal indications. This can lead to indications for use of the appropriate drug prepared homeopathically on a tautopathic indication to counteract the adverse effects of the conventional form of the drug. The potential detrimental influence of the use of the conventional preparations must not be underestimated, nor the time for which such influence may persist, especially if there is a miasmatic predisposition. Even though the administration of a particular agent has ceased well in the past, the use of that agent as a homeopathic preparation should always be considered as part of the treatment.

Many conditions involving the endocrine system are best approached from the constitutional point of view, and the major polychrests will feature largely among the remedies employed. The endocrine malfunction may also be part of a wider clinical picture that is tackled by way of a deep-seated approach. It must always be remembered that many endocrine imbalances can be improved by administration of the correct constitutional remedy. In some cases presented for homeopathic treatment the animal will already be receiving replacement therapy. This must not be withdrawn precipitously, but a close monitoring of the ensuing hormone levels must be undertaken and appropriate dosage adjustments made.

Major Modalities and Rubrics

Because of the widespread influence of the endocrine system on the body, rubrics reflecting its action are to be found throughout the repertory. The rubrics are mainly couched in terms of the effects of endocrine malfunction, with no direct mention of the gland involved. Even in those repertories that do not follow the Kentian format, only occasional references will be found to named endocrine conditions. Repertorisation in the classical manner, concentrating on the signs in the individual rather than the diagnosis, will yield the best results.

References to the direct consequences of hormonal malfunction of the reproductive systems will be found in the chapters devoted to those systems, i.e. male and female genital, where there are rubrics such as 'Menses; –absent, –prolonged, –profuse', etc. The functional similarity between 'oestrus' and 'menses' means that these rubrics can be used in animals. The effects of normal sexual hormonal activity on the rest of the body will be found under 'Generals', with > or < during the various stages of the menses. Physical changes to glands, when recorded, are to be found in the chapters that relate to the anatomical area in which the gland is located. However, the majority of endocrine upsets involve malfunction rather than pathology, and generally the useful rubrics represent the manifestations of that malfunction. Thus diabetes mellitus will be found in Kentian repertories via rubrics such as 'Urine; sugar', 'Stomach; thirst, extreme', 'Generals; emaciation', etc., which represent the picture as presented in a particular case. Headings of 'Diabetes Mellitus' in other repertories represent in the main a composite of such rubrics. However, it must be remembered that such rubrics are biased more towards common symptoms and do not contain any of the mental or other individualising features of a case. Allowance must also be made for the fact that a condition may present slightly differently in animals to humans.

Hormonal problems may well involve changes in the hair, particularly loss, and here the rubrics of 'Hair; falling' in both the Head and Skin chapters can be of use.

Remedies of Major Use

Calcarea Carbonica

The constitutional type here tends to be slow and placid. The physical conformation is usually large with heavy bones and a tendency to obesity. They are often lazy with weakness and lack of stamina. The slowness is a feature of all aspects of the type and involves both the physical movements and the metabolism. There is also slowness in the development of the young, with delayed dentition, etc. They are basically docile but can have fears and anxieties, together with an obstinate streak. This, together with their lack of initiative and curiosity makes them home-loving animals. They are chilly, due to their slow metabolism, and they will seek heat. The picture has many similarities with hypothyroidism and the remedy is often required in connection with thyroid problems.

Iodum

This remedy has an affinity with all glandular tissue, and many of the indications of Iodum and salts that contain it are concerned with conditions that involve the glandular systems of the body. It is perhaps the least heat-tolerant remedy in homeopathy and consequently the modality of < heat is a strong characteristic. At the same time there is a < damp. Animals are very active and always 'on the go'. Although there is not much frank fear there is an underlying anxiety in the type. There is usually marked emaciation, often in spite of a good, even ravenous appetite. Muscle weakness is seen in many cases. The coat can appear to be of poor quality, even in otherwise normal animals.

The remedy picture and the tissue affinity both point to its connection with the thyroid gland. Both under- and over-active thyroids may benefit from its use. Conditions involving the pancreas may also require it, and its use in ovarian problems should not be forgotten. With all glands, cases of both hyper- and hypo-function may require it.

Medorrhinum

This is the nosode of the gonorrhoeal infection and represents the sycotic miasm. There is thus a close connection generally between this remedy and the reproductive system, which includes the ovaries and testes. There is an excess of function with increased discharges which are often strong-smelling and tend to stain materials with which they come into contact.

Natrum Muriaticum

Because of its connection with water, and the tendency that it has towards retention, this remedy has indications in those conditions where upset of the fluid balance is a feature. Situations where the action of conventional medications which upset that balance, such as steroids, needs to be counteracted may call for its use, in addition to those other conditions with more primary upsets. It may prove useful in both Addison's and Cushing's disease.

Emaciation during, and slow recovery from, illness are a feature that may be a reflection of an endocrine involvement. The weight loss seen in hyperthyroidism can be a reflection of one aspect of the Natrum Muriaticum picture

Sepia

Conditions following neutering of mature animals of either sex will often benefit from Sepia. The picture of Sepia contains a lack of interest in sex and low libido, as well as the general sluggishness and stasis. Hence the remedy will often help the animal that slows down and puts on weight following neutering. The presenting picture, however, may well contain features that do not apparently fit the picture, but the aetiology is an important consideration in these cases.

Other Remedies to Consider

ACTH in potency
  Depression
  Irregular sexual function. Impotence in males
  Polydipsia and frequent micturition
  Dryness and irritation of the skin

Aristolochia Clematitis
  Strong aetiology of never well since use of chemical contraceptives
  Seasons shorter than normal or absent
  Vulval irritation. Brown discharges

Carcinosin
  Can act to generally normalise the endocrine function
  History of cancer in patient or family. Aetiology of vaccination
  Loves thunder and fireworks
  Loves chocolate to excess
  Reacts to seaside, and may be < or >

Syzygium Jambolanum
  Glucose in urine
  Polydipsia. Much urine with high specific gravity
  Weakness and emaciation
  Dry membranes of the mouth.
  Hormonal preparations in potency

Thyroidinum
  Emaciation and muscular weakness
  Rapid, weak pulse
  Desires cold water
  Frequent micturition. Albumin and glucose in urine
  Dry skin

Reference

Julian, O.A. (1979) *Materia Medica of New Homoeopathic Remedies.*
Beaconsfield: Beaconsfield Publishers.

Chapter 27

The Skin

General Considerations

In Paragraph 202 of the *Organon*, Hahnemann stresses the importance of treating the underlying imbalance of the vital force, rather than annihilating the symptoms by topical means. Denied this superficial expression of disease, the vital force awakens the remaining, internal, symptoms of the disease, which had previously remained dormant. This phenomenon is generally referred to as 'suppression' but as can be seen from Hahnemann's explanation, the term is not strictly accurate; it is nevertheless the description used by the majority of homeopaths, and as long as the true mechanism of the observed effects is understood it is acceptable to use this definition. The dangers of suppression as thus defined are, however, those that demand that skin disease is treated correctly. The use of topical agents such as corticosteroids and the surgical removal of skin lesions are therefore contraindicated from a homeopathic point of view, but of far greater import is the use of systemic anti-inflammatory drugs. While antibiotics and antifungal agents seem to be less suppressive, their continued use is counterproductive; if the correct homeopathic medicine is administered they should become unnecessary. That being said, every patient is an individual, with their own individual strength of vital force, and an animal with low vital force may exhibit symptoms of overwhelming or deep-seated infection, such as deep furunculosis or massive burdens of malassezia. In such a case the strategic use of systemic antibiotics or topical antifungal agents can act synergistically with homeopathic medicine by lifting the energetic burden sufficiently to allow the vital force to react. This situation is, however, rare.

The effects of homeopathic suppression as predicted by Hahnemann are easily observed in veterinary practice. Firstly the symptoms recur, and at increasingly short intervals; secondly when they do recur, they are more severe; and thirdly, eventually, the deeper organs are affected. It may be pertinent at this point to reassess from a homeopathic point of view the progression of an atopic dog treated with corticosteroids towards steroid dependency, iatrogenic Cushing's disease and hepatic, renal or cardiac failure. On the subject of atopy, the other major factor which must be considered when treating homeopathically is that of vaccination, and it is the authors' experience that to continue the annual vaccination of an atopic animal is to render homeopathic treatment almost completely ineffective. Vaccinations almost invariably aggravate the skin symptoms of these patients, sometimes irreparably, and the importance of this issue in the context of the homeopathic treatment of skin diseases cannot be overstressed.

Sadly, many of the patients who are presented for homeopathic treatment of skin diseases are in an advanced state; in addition they frequently have histories of long-term suppressive therapy, often still in process. The effect of the latter is to bury signs of the true homeopathic disease, along with the animal's mental and general characteristics, under a fog of non-specific symptomatology, so much so that it is frequently impossible to see any clear constitutional picture. It is most important with such patients to 'hasten slowly', and in these cases the use of 'clearing remedies' such as bowel nosodes or miasmatic nosodes is to be recommended for initial prescriptions. Indeed, in his later life, Hahnemann himself frequently used Sulphur as an initial prescription in patients suffering from chronic disease, apparently on the basis of its power as a clearing remedy. Such medicines have the effect of 'clearing the picture' and allow a more accurate prescription to be made at follow-up. In addition, identifying the predominant miasm is a major step in successful treatment of skin disease and to that end the table opposite should be of assistance.

The suppressive effects of corticosteroids may persevere for weeks or months after administration has ceased, and tautopathic treatment with potentised corticosteroid may help to remove them more rapidly. It should be noted that the homeopathic proving of cortisone (by Templeton, described in *Materia Medica of New Homoeopathic Remedies* by Julian) produces symptoms indistinguishable from allergic dermatitis, and in cases of longstanding steroid therapy, sometimes all that is required is a course of potentised cortisone, prednisolone or other such corticosteroid as may be appropriate for the case.

In allergies, the isopathic use of potentised allergens, identified by skin or blood testing, may prove a useful adjunct to more classical prescriptions, but it should again be borne in mind that this does not address the underlying imbalance in the vital force and can at best be

A Miasmatic Classification of Skin Diseases

Psora	Sycosis	Syphilis	Tuberculosis
Dry	Warty	Ulcers	Pustules
Rough	Circumscribed	Flexures of limbs	Smooth
Spreads	Localised		History of ringworm
Itch	Pain	Pus, blood	
Dirty	Oily	Offensive	Urticaria
Scales thin	Pigment changes	Scales thick	Obstinate boils
		Glandular swelling	Glandular swelling

Effects of suppression			
Mind	Reproductive	Meninges (paralysis)	Deeper tissues
CNS	Liver	Eyes	Suppuration
Colitis	Heart	Bones	Cavitation

palliative. In this context, a vaccine composed of allergens is no different from any other vaccine in the way it affects the vital force, and the repeated insults to the immune system which such vaccination regimes involve seem to render the organism extremely refractory to homeopathy.

On the subject of ectoparasites, the increased level of general health, coupled with the improved immune response which can occur with homeopathic treatment, may be sufficient for an animal to throw off such a burden. Sometimes, however, the vital force does not seem to be able to respond sufficiently. In addition, the continued irritation caused by the parasites constitutes an obstacle to cure, and in these cases removal by some other, topical, means is necessary.

Ear problems are treated homeopathically in the same way as skin disease, reflecting the fact that the ear canal is lined by modified skin. However, the shape of the canine ear in particular renders its aeration and drainage highly critical, and anything further affecting this delicate balance sends the external ear into a downward spiral of swelling of the ear canal, increased secretion, decreased aeration and decreased drainage. In such circumstances homeopathy can still bring about remarkable improvements in otitis externa, but frequently some topical treatment is necessary, such as flushing with Calendula lotion. Occasionally some conventional medication is still required to bring about total resolution of the problem, but if this is so, the response to the conventional medicine when used alongside homeopathy may be expected to be superior to that when it is used alone.

In line with homeopathic philosophy, the mental and emotional state of the patient is of immense importance in the development of skin disease, and in cats it is paramount; feline skin disease almost invariably has its cause rooted deeply in the emotional sphere, and its successful homeopathic treatment depends on identifying the change in the animal's routine or home environment which has triggered it. While this is of equal importance in dogs, it is in the feline species that the emotional cause can often be more readily identified.

Homeopathic treatment of skin diseases can therefore be complex, and in chronic disease patience is required by veterinary surgeon and client; for instance, it often takes three seasons for total resolution of atopy. However, the rewards are great, and it is for this reason that skin disease represents a major part of the caseload in homeopathic referral practice. Not all patients presented with skin disease respond to homeopathy, but with patience and perseverance it is uncommon to find one who will not benefit in some way from homeopathic medicine.

Finally, the inevitable note on diet. There is no doubt that patients suffering from skin disease will benefit from a diet based on whole raw foods such as those already mentioned; of particular importance are the essential fatty acids, and the one simple dietary measure above all others which will benefit these patients is the addition of cold-pressed hempseed, flaxseed or fish oil to the food.

Major Modalities and Rubrics

In the repertory, the key word for skin lesions is 'eruptions'. There is a whole section of the repertory devoted to the skin, but the location of lesions in the patient is also important to note, and for this reference must be made to the appropriate anatomical section. 'Axilla' will be found under 'Chest', and 'Inguinal' under 'Abdomen'. 'Chin' will be found under 'Face'.

The appearance of the skin will include thickening and change in colour, and the lesions ('eruptions') may be classified as to whether they are discharging, desquamating, circinate, vesicular, pustular and so on. Warts and tumours may also be noted, either in the general 'Skin' section or the appropriate location.

Due to anatomical differences, using human repertories is problematical when it comes to greasiness of the coat in animals; however, using the rubrics 'Perspiration; oily' or 'Face; greasy' seems to be a valid approach, though the authors' preference is for the latter.

Perhaps more important than the appearance of the lesions are the modalities and sensations, as these are a more specific response to the energetic imbalance. In an animal which is scratching it seems reasonable to assume the presence of pruritus, and in practice the rubric 'itching' and its sub-rubrics can certainly be used with confidence. Such factors as the effect of heat and cold, bathing, open air and movement can be extremely useful, as can the time modalities. Where the specific skin rubrics are not reliable, recourse can be made to the Generalities. The response to itching in animals is usually to scratch the affected area, and the effect of this may be to cause bleeding, or rawness. Sometimes the scratching aggravates the itch; at other times it ameliorates it; at yet other times it causes the itch to change places.

Constitutional prescriptions will bring about the most lasting improvements in patients suffering from skin disease, and a vital piece of information in this identification is the general heat modality of the animal. A very chilly animal, or a very hot one, can immediately be categorised into a smaller number of possible homeopathic remedies, and it is well worth the extra time it may take in a consultation to gain an accurate picture of the heat modalities of the patient.

Remedies of Major Use

Sulphur

Sulphur has a deserved reputation in skin disease, and just about every skin lesion imaginable is found in its materia medica. In consequence, the nondescript symptomatology presented in many cases of chronic skin disease means that repertorisation almost invariably indicates Sulphur. However, despite the vagueness of the symptoms this medicine is frequently useful in such cases. In low potency it has a very useful non-specific effect on the skin, and advantage may be taken of this by using it to wean an animal off corticosteroids – for example,

Sulphur 6c may be given b.i.d. concurrent with gradually reducing the dosage of the steroids. Once this process is complete a clearer homeopathic picture should be available to the prescriber. If the symptomatology still suggests Sulphur, then a higher potency may be used. However, it is prudent to note that Sulphur in higher potency, given to a patient who has been suppressed for some time, may result in severe aggravation, so caution should be exercised here.

The skin lesions of Sulphur are classically dry, red and itchy and affect mainly the trunk, but other common sites include the feet and around the eyes. The itch is made worse by heat in any form, particularly the heat of the bed, so affected animals frequently start to itch a few minutes after they have settled down in their bed or basket. Bathing, too aggravates. Other lesions include moist dermatitis, pustular eruptions and excoriations in folds of the skin. There may be desquamation and the skin and coat look dirty, with an offensive musty smell. Scratching often ameliorates, so the animal scratches only intermittently; at other times it only aggravates the situation so that raw, discharging or bloody lesions occur.

The skin of Sulphur is generally unhealthy, so wounds heal slowly and are prone to secondary infection.

The ears of Sulphur are red and itchy, and exude an offensive mucopurulent discharge.

As a first prescription for many patients with skin disease, Sulphur can be highly beneficial; and especially where the disease is chronic, the keynotes of 'hot, itchy and smelly' are enough to justify its prescription. If this can be further matched to the mental and general symptoms of Sulphur described earlier, then the effects will be correspondingly more profound.

Arsenicum Album

With Arsenicum there is virtually always some desquamation; white flakes of dandruff accompany intense itching. Patients often scratch till they bleed, and continued scratching leads to chronic thickening of the skin and the so-called 'elephant hide' appearance. Bright red blotches may appear on the skin, especially on the chest and abdomen; there may also be vesicles, pimples or ulcers. Ear discharges tend to be thin and excoriating. The itch is characteristically worse after midnight, and for this reason owners often complain that the dog scratches all night and disturbs their sleep. Aggravation of itching may occur in cold damp weather and by the seaside, and the seasonal periodicity of Arsenicum is a reminder of the value of Arsenicum in atopy. Finally, a reminder of the heat modalities of Arsenicum; these patients sit almost on top of the fire, beside the central heating boiler, or right up against a radiator, and they will bake in the sun. This extreme chilliness, along with the white dandruff and nightly aggravation, can lead one rapidly into considering Arsenicum; confirmation should then be sought by investigating more mental and general symptoms.

Natrum Muriaticum

Natrum Mur. has alopecia and greasiness of the coat; skin lesions tend to be symmetrical and there is some predilection for the bends of the limbs. In humans, herpetic eruptions around the mouth come within its remit, and in animals this is reflected by the presence of crusty lesions around the mouth and in the corners of the lips. The classic human symptom of a crack in the middle of the lower lip is occasionally seen in animals. The greasiness of the coat leads to easy matting, and occasionally the hair may stick together in the 'paintbrush' lesions reminiscent of rain scald in horses. Again, there is dandruff of white flakes.

Specific lesions may be vesicular, crusty, or moist; there may also be red patches or urticarial swellings.

Natrum Mur. is one of the most commonly successful remedies for treating miliary dermatitis in cats, especially where grief can be identified as a causative factor.

The itching of Nat. Mur. is better for cool bathing, may be better – or worse – at the seaside, and tends to be worse for heat. There may be a periodicity where symptoms are worse on alternate days.

Pulsatilla Nigricans

The skin lesions of Pulsatilla are classically described as 'measly'. Vesicles rapidly turn to crusts and these are often distributed widely over the abdomen, extending to the genitals and sometimes down the back legs. The rest of the trunk may also be affected and, less commonly, the limbs, although there may be itching of the feet. Itching is worse for heat and worse in the evenings. Gentle motion in the open air relieves the itch and rubbing also ameliorates, so the preferred method of dealing with the itch is for the patient to rub herself along the floor. Pulsatilla is also a medicine for recurring urticaria, especially where it is made worse by heat and exertion (this, incidentally, is the opposite of Sepia).

The right ear is more severely affected than the left, and discharges tend to be purulent, often green to yellow but mainly bland. Otitis media may occur. Pulsatilla is also often indicated in miliary dermatitis.

Rhus Toxicodendron

Rhus Tox. (American Poison Ivy) causes a red, vesicular rash which is intensely itchy. This is similar to that of Pulsatilla, but the itching is more intense and the vesicular stage is more readily apparent; sometimes this is seen as a 'cobbled' appearance to the skin, especially noticeable over the hindquarters. With Rhus Tox., the itch is so intense as to cause the animal to pull all the hair out of the region affected, and then to continue to scratch and bite at the area until it is raw and bleeding. Occasionally the area may become moist as a result. The itching is worse at night, particularly in bed, and there is a characteristic aggravation in the morning in bed; once the patient is up and moving, the itch is relieved. Covering may also ameliorate the itching and this can be determined by dressing a pruritic dog in a T-shirt. In humans the itching is relieved by bathing in scalding hot water but this has not been observed in animals by the authors!

Where there has been prolonged scratching, the skin becomes thickened and discoloured.

Itching around the eyes and of the eyelids causes rubbing and consequent alopecia and excoriation in this area.

The pinna may show similar lesions to the skin elsewhere, and there may be an associated chronic otitis externa with sanguinopurulent discharge.

Mentally these patients are often bright, cheerful and good-humoured and it is certainly the happy-go-lucky terrier which seems to develop a Rhus Tox. skin more than any other type.

Other Remedies to Consider

Graphites
  Sticky, honey-coloured discharges
  Lesions in skin folds, esp. interdigital, axilla, groin
  Patient is fat, chilly and lazy

Ignatia Amara
  Obsessive licking – lick granuloma, interdigital dermatitis
  Skin eruptions like nettle-rash
  History of grief or separation

Mercurius Solubilis
 Wet dermatitis; lesions purulent, smelly, green
 Otitis externa with foul-smelling discharges of pus and blood
 Patient is thirsty with wet mouth

Staphysagria
 Itchy, scabby lesions all over body; miliary dermatitis in cats
 Itching changes place on scratching
 History of surgery or other emotional upset

Thuja Occidentalis
 Thickening, pigmentation
 Warts, especially on perineum or genitalia
 History of vaccination

References

Banerjea, S.K. (1993) *Miasmatic Diagnosis.* New Delhi: B. Jain Publishers Ltd.
Julian, O.A. (1979) *Materia Medica of New Homoeopathic Remedies.* Beaconsfield: Beaconsfield Publishers.

Chapter 28

Behavioural Problems

General Considerations

The mind and the body are intimately linked and it is recognised in the human field that emotional disturbance, if not properly addressed, can lead on to physical manifestations of disease. It is said that 'the body sheds the tears the eyes cannot weep', implying that it is in the suppression of emotions and normal behaviour patterns that the roots of many troubles lie. Because of the pervading culture of human dominance in relation to animals it is easy to forget that they too can be similarly affected.

One thing to consider is that what an owner describes as a behavioural problem may in fact be the animal reacting normally to a situation. Problems are usually defined in terms of human social parameters. A cat that begins to spray in the house may well be producing the normal response of the species to a changed situation. This may be the introduction of a new animal into the household causing, from the cat's point of view, a change in the pack dynamics. Treatment with homeopathy will concentrate on identifying the mental change in the cat, i.e. fear, resentment, rejection, etc. and basing the remedy selection on that. In contrast, conventional medication aims at controlling the situation by adjusting the hormones. Not only is it less successful (Chapter 2), but because it has not addressed the root of the problem the mental disturbance is still there and the seeds of future ill health may be being laid.

Because of the difficulties in identifying the thought processes of animals, the effects of these are often underrated. Although perhaps not all the shades of emotions that are seen in humans are present in animals, nevertheless many are. The more basic emotions of fear etc. are easily observed and give rise to some of the behavioural problems that are seen. Many, however, such as grief, are not and can only be inferred. This is where the inclusion of the social history in case taking is so important, not only for providing the vital clues in behavioural problems, but also for providing the key to many physical conditions.

It is also essential to understand the normal social patterns of the individual species in order to appreciate fully when and how human expectations and actions affect them. For example, budgerigars, together with other avian species, are naturally gregarious, living in large colonies, whereas in domestication they are often kept either singly or in small groups. In these circumstances, the interactions with their human companions may be vitally important for their wellbeing, as substitutes for the natural flock. Consequently any upsets in these interactions can have profound effects. Similarly, a school pet such as a hamster, removed for the holidays from the activity and attention of the classroom to the quieter environment of a private home, may suffer an emotional upset. The loss of freedom inherent in the zoological situation can on occasion, no matter how good the management, trigger problems in those species whose natural lifestyle is of a nomadic nature.

Some behavioural changes, of course, arise from a physical condition, and these must be recognised as such. Similarly, old age brings its own changes. These and possible remedies are discussed in Chapter 29.

Many animals are placed in situations that are alien to their natural tendencies, and are asked to perform tasks which are only of relevance to their owners. This applies not only in relation to showing and performing, but also to the commercial requirements of food production. The expected behavioural standards in these situations are entirely those of the owners, however much they may be justified by the 'he enjoys it' type of rationalisation. Domestication has certainly produced an amazing degree of adaptation and acquiescence on the part of all species. Nevertheless it must be remembered that the criteria by which much behaviour is judged have been established entirely from the human point of view. An animal may be behaving perfectly rationally according to its own standards and still not meet these criteria. The human demands for activities which the animal would not necessarily undertake in nature (e.g. dressage and showing), linked to the high expectations of the handlers, can lead to the creation of a state of high control and limitation being imposed on the animal. This may lead to the creation of particular remedy states, such as Carcinosin, which has the control pattern in its picture together with the expectation of high performance. This situation may indicate a prescription on an aetiological basis.

In the treatment of genuine behavioural problems the higher potencies will usually be required. If possible, of course, removal of the cause should be undertaken although in many cases this will not be feasible. A realisation of the true emotional needs of the animal is essential, and it may be possible to alter the environment in ways that are acceptable to the humans concerned while at the same time meeting the needs of other species.

Some behavioural problems are examples of what Hahnemann calls 'one-sided diseases'. In these the symptom picture is of one predominating feature, and as a consequence the finding of the simillimum becomes more difficult. In such a case removal of the presenting mental symptom can act as a form of suppression and ultimately result in the development of more physically-based problems. While such suppression most commonly occurs as a result of conventional medication it must not be forgotten that homeopathy is also capable of being used in a suppressive manner. For example, if Belladonna is used continuously to control the onset of aggressive behaviour in a cat, this may well mask the fact that the reason for the aggression, in the form of resentment at the arrival of another cat, is not being addressed. Hence the resentment will be suppressed and will find its outlet in another direction. In presenting a behavioural case at the consultation, owners' usual tendencies to concentrate on what they perceive as the problem often reaches its highest pitch, as there are often social dimensions to the situation. Thus it is vital to bear this in mind, and explore all other aspects of the animal's health and history to try and broaden the prescribing base as much as possible.

In some cases of vaccinosis the initial presenting picture can be purely on the mental and emotional level.

The manifestation of mental disease (which is what behavioural problems are), will always involve a degree of loss of control and thus, from the miasmatic point of view, there is always a strong psoric influence in mental disease. However, the initial treatment should not be with predominantly anti-psoric remedies. The other influences must be eliminated first, with the psoric picture emerging as the final stage before cure.

It must be remembered that homeopathy can only optimalise behaviour, not create or maintain abnormal patterns. Homeopathy is about re-establishing natural patterns. Continuous imposition of abnormal behaviour patterns will constitute an obstacle to cure and in these circumstances all that can be achieved is a degree of alleviation.

Major Modalities and Rubrics

The mind section of the repertory is that most needed with behavioural problems. The 'Never Well Since' approach can be extremely useful in these cases and hence the rubrics of 'ailments from' are important. The section on delusions should not be ignored, although it must be interpreted with care. Animals that suddenly turn and snap at some empty space behind their shoulder may have the delusion that there is someone hovering just behind them (part of the Medorrhinum picture). As discussed above, other symptoms should be included wherever possible, and general symptoms are the most fruitful area to explore.

The major emotions that effect animals are:

- Grief – This includes loneliness and self-pity.

- Anger – This incorporates resentment.

- Love – There are relevant rubrics here. Possessiveness and jealousy are part of this.

- Hate/fear/anxiety – Stress and tension usually show as these. Stress can also show as an inability to cope, with various types of displacement behaviour being manifest. Lick granulomata can arise in this way, or patterns of destructive behaviour.

The timing of the observed behavioural reactions may give clues to the underlying factors, such as changes in behaviour linked to the appearance or disappearance of particular individuals, or the onset being linked to a set time of day when something is happening in the environment on a regular basis. It must also be remembered that there are differences in the range and intensity of the senses in the various species, and this will influence the interpretation of rubrics produced from human experience. Care must also be taken over the use of rubrics that have an entirely different connotation in humans to that seen in animals. For example, yawning in pack animals is part of the communication techniques that ensure peaceful co-existence, which is entirely different to the physiological reaction behind the rubric interpreting human reactions. In the repertory, rubrics linked to yawning are found in the chapters 'Cough', 'Sleep' and 'Generals', whereas the 'Mind' section would be the appropriate place if the phenomenon was part of the social interaction of the species. Similarly, horses that whinny excessively are often exhibiting anxiety or fear, rather than 'loquacity' as found in the repertory.

Remedies of Major Use

Argentum Nitricum

This is one of the great remedies for anticipatory anxiety and fear, which may manifest as bowel symptoms with diarrhoea and flatulence. The nervousness will also produce much trembling and limb weakness. There are often irrational fears and animals may refuse to follow a certain route for no apparent reason. As would be expected, there is a desire for company, and solitude can produce destructive behaviour or self-mutilation. One particular fear is of high places, and also of high buildings falling onto them. This is translated in animals into an aversion to being approached from above by vets, show judges and so on. Together with the anticipatory fear of 'performing', this makes it one of the leading remedies for behavioural problems associated with showing. One of the paradoxes of the remedy is that in spite of the fear there is often a compulsion to seek danger, and an impulsiveness in the movements.

Ignatia

The main action of Ignatia is on the mind and the nervous system, and the overwhelming reaction is cramping on both the emotional and physical levels. There is a high degree of hypersensitivity generally in the picture, with a low pain threshold. Changes of mood are a feature, and although there is an unpredictability the animal is not intrinsically aggressive. There is depression with much yawning and sighing, which also gives much neighing, whining, etc. It is a contradictory remedy and can give unexpected reactions – a desire for indigestible items which are eaten with no ill effects, or a sore throat which is > swallowing solids but < swallowing liquids.

The major aetiologies of Ignatia are mental – ailments from fright, anticipation, grief, and similar emotions. Separation from loved ones, especially a parent, is very marked. Ignatia is often indicated when the emotional event is in the recent past. Although this is not an absolute rule, the longer ago the trigger and the more pathology there is associated with the condition, the more Natrum Muriaticum will be indicated.

The functional upsets involve spasms. These may involve whole muscle groups with loss or impaired use of the limbs. Alternatively there may be twitching of muscles, especially around the face, with tossing of the head backwards. There is much twitching of the limbs during sleep. Another form of spasm that may be seen is convulsions.

Lachesis

The major modality of this remedy is < suppressed discharges and this has implications in the mental sphere resulting in behavioural changes prior to oestrus. There is also the opposite modality of > for discharges starting to flow. Another marked feature is an aggravation from sleep. Jealousy is marked in the picture and undesirable reactions as a result of this will often respond. There is an aggression that can on occasion become hysterical. There is a general air of nervous energy surrounding a Lachesis animal with quick movements, restlessness, and sensitivity to all impressions. Great loquacity is also a feature and this shows as the animal that barks, growls or moans incessantly and will not stop when told to. Some animals will be antisocial and seek to be alone. An upset in the sense of time occurs, with restless behaviour at night.

Lachesis is a valuable tool in the treatment of the ill effects of rabies vaccination. Following vaccination many animals will develop an intense irritation around the base of the tail which can be aggravated by self-mutilation. In the Lachesis picture there is an inflammation of the meninges in the region of the coccyx causing such an intense irritation. There is also a fear of and dislike for water, which gives another connection to rabies, with its hydrophobia.

Natrum Muriaticum

On the mental level both sodium and chlorine are concerned with relationships. Sodium is concerned with the making, or failure to make relationships, chlorine is more concerned with the ending of relationships.

The aetiology of behavioural problems requiring Nat. Mur. is thus often centred around the loss of companions, both animal and human. Mental trauma in any form may call for its use, but especially where grief or rejection are involved.

One theme that runs through Nat. Mur. on both the mental and physical levels is that of retention. On the physical level this shows as conditions involving retention of fluids and upset to the fluid balance in the body. Mentally the Nat. Mur. animal rarely forgets and never forgives. Following a mental hurt the overwhelming impulse is to avoid getting into situations where they can be hurt again. They hence become loners, and this is the basis of the modality < consolation. The paradox is that underneath they want to be loved, and so their behaviour can be friendly and playful up to a point, but beyond that they change. They can be 'nice to know, hell to live with', with sudden and unpredictable aggression, and they can be irritable, nervous, and angry.

This picture fits many dogs and cats that have been through stray kennels, and horses that have been sold to new owners and undergo a temperament change.

Apart from the aggression that is often shown in these situations, these animals will appear depressed and withdrawn. They appear not to know how to play, or will indulge in bursts of hysterical activity.

The aloof and independent nature of many cats makes the remedy one that is of major use in the species.

There is an aversion to sex in the picture and this shows in the animal that will actively and aggressively resist mating.

Staphysagria

Sensitivity, anger and resentment are the basis of the mental picture here. There is sensitivity to all 'insults', whether mental or physical, but the anger and resentment tend to be bottled up. Although there is often an apparent gentleness in the picture, when the anger does come out it takes the form of a violent outburst. There is a modality < wounds with sharp object. Tissues are also particularly affected by being stretched. Hence its use in animals that are depressed and healing poorly after surgery.

One area of affinity is with the urogenital system. Idiopathic cystitis may respond if there is a mental connection. Spraying in neutered cats following an upset in the balance of their environment can be successfully treated with the remedy. Many cases of so-called flea allergic dermatitis in neutered cats will also respond.

Other Remedies to Consider

Aconite
  Sudden shocks and onset of fear. Can be used on a 'Never Well Since' basis
  Full rapid pulse
  Great restlessness
  Hysteria from fear

Belladonna
  Sudden onset
  Aggression
  Unsteady gait and tendency to fall. Head shaking
  Full, bounding pulse. Dilated pupils
  Hallucinations and convulsions

Hyoscyamus
  Twitching of facial muscles. May be distortion of expression
  Convulsions. Vertigo before attack. Animal screams and falls
  Excessive licking of genitals
  Exhibitionist behaviour. Lewd in humans

Nux Vomica
  Anger and impatience
  Sensitive to external stimuli. Low pain threshold
  Tendency take everything to excess. Moves quickly
  Fearful, especially in males

Tuberculinum
  Discontented. Always wanting something different
  Easily bored with same food
  Changeable symptoms
  Fits of anger. Will resent discipline (Bacillinum)
  Sensitive to noise

Reference

Scholten, J. (1996) *Homeopathy and the Elements*. Utrecht, The Netherlands: Stichting Alonnissos.

Chapter 29

The Geriatric Patient

General Considerations

It must be remembered that ageing itself is not a disease in the conventional sense. It is a progressive and normal reduction of the ability to maintain homeostasis in the face of physiological and external stresses. The elderly pet is seldom afflicted with a single condition but rather with varying degrees of multi-organ and system dysfunction. There is a decreased *ability* to maintain the balance that we call health. In homeopathic terms, this can easily become a situation of 'dis-ease', but it is important to decide whether the symptoms are part of the ageing process or represent the progression of genuine chronic disease.

One consequence of this loss of homeostatic ability is an increased susceptibility to disease in the conventional sense. However, when confronted by such a case it must always be borne in mind that there is this underlying difficulty in maintaining balance that must be considered as well as the more acute picture.

There is inevitably a weakening of the vital force with age. But this can be to a very variable degree, and age of itself does not imply a very low vital force. If an animal has had a basically healthy life, with little disease or antagonistic medication, then the major effects on the system will be the normal wear and tear of time. There will be a certain loss of both tissue and function in the vital organs, and when this becomes critical enough the physiological balance cannot be maintained. The function of homeopathic remedies in these cases is to help in restoring and maintaining that balance. But the vital force, although weakening with age, may be stronger than at first thought, and hence capable of responding to a more vigorous stimulus. On the other hand, in an animal with a long and involved medical history, chronic disease and advanced pathology will often be present. Homeopathically, advanced pathology is an indication of a weakened vital force, and the force may have been extensively weakened along the way. Hence in old age it will require the gentler stimulus of lower potencies, even with well-selected remedies. Other manifestations of chronic disease will also point to the use of

278

lower potencies. But do not assume that the lower potencies are always the only ones that will be needed in older animals, as some patients will be able to respond to a stronger stimulus. There are also cases where successful treatment will lead to a strengthening of the vital force to some degree.

When considering the medical history, it must be borne in mind that what are conventionally regarded as safe, routine, and desirable preventative procedures can have detrimental effects on the body. Overuse of vaccines, flea treatments (especially systemic), wormers, etc. can upset the vital balance. This effect is magnified if the overuse of these agents is continued into old age.

It must also be accepted that a control and maintenance situation is often all that can be achieved, rather than a cure. This can result in the sort of prolonged dosage regimes that would not be considered in other circumstances. This may seem at first sight to be merely palliation, and in certain circumstances this may be desirable from the welfare point of view as being all that can be achieved. However, there will be cases in which there is a more curative action. In all cases it is important to remember to let the patient show the prescriber what potency and frequency of administration is needed, rather than any assumptions being made that result in overdosage.

One of the consequences of the ageing process is a progressive reduction in metabolic rate. This has relevance in the selection of potency and in the assessment of the response to treatment. Lower potencies may be required to provide a more gentle stimulus to the vital force, but if higher potencies are used their action may persist for longer. It must be remembered that it also has an effect on the utilisation and elimination of conventional medication. There is a tendency for the half-life of drugs to increase in the old patient.

There are two conditions that are particularly associated with increasing age. One is neoplasia. The incidence of neoplasia rises with age, but many will be benign. Although the overall incidence is higher in the dog than the cat, there is a higher incidence of malignancy in the latter (Wills and Wolf). The advisability or otherwise of removal must be carefully considered, even in cases of known malignancy. The risks of anaesthesia etc. apart, removal on its own can be a form of suppression and may result in the appearance of more aggressive neoplasia in a more vital organ. This tendency may be reversed by the administration of the appropriate constitutional or miasmatic remedy. The likely rate of growth of a neoplasm in the older animal must also be considered when assessing the justification for removal.

The cardiovascular incident (CVI), also known as the geriatric vestibular syndrome (GVS) is the other condition of age. In animals this not the true 'stroke' of human medicine, with the associated blocking of vessels, although these do occur. The aetiology is unclear, and it appears to be more of a transient ischaemic attack. Increase in blood pressure may produce the symptoms. Although blood pressure rises with age it has been shown in the dog that, in the absence of other disease, the rise is less than is seen in man.

Major Modalities and Rubrics

One of the areas in which the effects of ageing are most apparent is that of behaviour. This may in part be secondary to loss of function of the senses, but there is a primary upset as well. This shows as decreased reaction to stimuli of all sorts, and a degree of confusion and disorientation. Increased vocalisation and alterations in the sleep/wake cycle can be particularly distressing for owners, and these are often the presenting symptoms. Compulsive behaviour and loss of previous learning also cause great concern. Animals may develop aggressive behaviour but this is usually linked to anxiety states. Loss of senses must be borne in mind when considering behavioural changes and modalities.

Thermoregulatory ability decreases with age, and this can affect the interpretation of heat modalities.

The normal uncomplicated process of ageing has a tendency towards thirst reduction.

However, rubrics involving thirst must be used with caution as ageing may involve an associated condition (e.g. renal disease) where thirst is a common symptom.

Relevant rubrics are to be found throughout the repertory, but direct references to age may not always be there. Thus incontinence without any link to age will be found under 'Bladder; urination; involuntary' only, and while there is a rubric for 'Bladder; urination; frequent; in old people' it is too small a rubric to be of much use.The chapter on Vertigo is probably of more use in geriatric prescribing than in any other area of veterinary work.

All modalities in age must be viewed within the general context of a decrease in reactivity.

Remedies of Major Use

Arnica

This is a remedy that has such a (deserved) reputation in the trauma situation that its other uses are often overlooked. It is an excellent remedy for general support of the muscular and cardiovascular systems. It will help to maintain muscle mass and tone. It also has indications in oedema and congestion of the respiratory system. Because of its action on both the cardiovascular and respiratory systems it has a major role in the management of heart conditions in the older animal. It is indicated in the cardiovascular incident syndrome (GVS) due to the vertigo that is present in the picture.

Haemorrhages of any origin may call for its use.

There is a great fear of being touched, and a constant bruised feeling. Conditions are < for exertion. The animal will show restlessness due to being < pressure, and the bed or ground always feel too hard. At the same time there is a desire to lie down, preferably on the right side. There is mental depression combined with physical restlessness.

Other symptoms are < injury, overexertion, touch, sleep, motion, damp cold, lying on left, > lying down, lying with head stretched out, motion. The remedy often has a general support role in many conditions affecting the geriatric patient. It can be used in addition to other indicated remedies, and in acute incidents.

Dosage here is in accordance with the general principles of more frequent administration in acute conditions and less frequent in chronic states.

The Baryta salts in general

These are possibly the single most useful group of remedies in the support of the geriatric patient. Their greatest use is at the extremes of life. There is a general tendency to bleeding and ulceration of the mouth, salivation, foul-smelling breath, and glandular enlargement.

The themes of the component elements of these salts cover the powerlessness, insecurity, degeneration, weakness and dependency that characterise this age group. Barium toxicity induces heart failure, degeneration of blood vessels, hypertension, lowering of blood potassium levels and muscular spasm followed by paralysis, all of which find their echo in the older animal. The anions show themes of dependency, loss of security, bereavement and rejection that are again met with in the extremes of life.

Baryta Carbonica

Emaciation with normal appetite.

General weakness of limbs with desire to lie down whenever possible.

Great dependency and anxiety.

Paralysis after CVI.

Senile dementia. Dullness. Timidity. Irrational barking.

Abdominal pain < eating. Sluggish rumination. Constipation.

Palpitations of the heart.

Perspiration at rest, not increased by movement. Sweat does not dry quickly.

< cold (chills), heat of sun, eating.

> warmth, motion.

Baryta Iodata

Hardening and opacity are its themes.

Weakness of memory. Dog will stand staring at nothing, or forget house training.

Emaciation.

Tumours involving lymph tissue. The mesenteric glands are often involved. Hard swellings.

< warmth, walking.

> cold, open air.

Baryta Muriatica

This is the barium salt that has the greatest action on the cardiovascular system.

There is also a tendency to convulsions and a general loss of muscular power.

Aneurysms feature in the picture. The pulse is either soft and irregular or full and rapid. There is a high systolic pressure with a low diastolic. Swings between these two causes collapse without loss of consciousness, and with rapid recovery.

< climbing, cold air, open air (but will seek it), morning. wet weather, autumn.

Baryta Sulphurica

Anxiety and suspicion.

Has a tendency to develop heart problems.

A right-sided remedy.

Pain in bones and stiffness in joints. Involuntary jerking of muscles with loss of muscle tone.

< exertion, cold, eating, morning.

> walking in open air.

Causticum

This is a potassium salt and has the weakness associated with the group. Muscular weakness will progress to paralysis of single parts. There is contraction of tendons, with stiffness and pain. The left hip may be particularly painful.

A general appearance of an 'old, broken-down animal'. Laryngeal and facial paralysis. Recurrent cystitis as a result of urinary retention. Faecal and urinary incontinence; faeces are passed involuntarily as animal is walking. Flat warts are seen, especially on the face. There is cardiac involvement with palpitations and pain. A dry cough that gives the impression that it would ease if only mucus could be expelled.

< dry cold, wind, extremes of temperature, exertion, entering a warm room, bathing.

> warmth of bed, damp wet weather, and paradoxically, cold dry weather.

Conium

'Ascending' is the word to remember in connection with Conium. There is ascending paralysis of the limbs which moves upwards from the feet, and the remedy often gives its best results when used in ascending potencies. Weakness of the hind legs, with trembling of muscles and sudden but temporary loss of strength within a picture of steady decline. It has uses in cases of tumours where the swellings are stony hard. Involuntary passage of motion while the animal is asleep is also seen.

< exertion, cold, night, standing, resting.

> moving, pressure, heat of sun.

Lycopodium

This is one of the great constitutional remedies. Its action involves most systems of the body but in the context of the geriatric animal the mental, alimentary, respiratory, urinary and musculoskeletal systems are all influenced. There is a gradual deterioration in all systems. Anxiety and mental weakness are seen. Indigestion occurs with great flatulence. Dyspnoea, cystitis and enlarged prostate are all features, as are stiffness and pain in muscles, often with marked sensitivity to pain. It is a right-sided remedy.

< eating, wind and draughts, 4-8 p.m., crowds, wet weather.
> motion, passing wind, urinating.

Other Remedies to Consider

Arsenicum Album
    Generally supports the older system, especially in cases of malignancy
    Gradual weight loss leading to emaciation
    Easy exhaustion after slight activity
    Feelings of anxiety and insecurity
    Ascites

Carbo Animalis
    Weakness of old age
    Venous stasis
    < loss of even small quantities of body fluids
    Failure to convalesce after illness

Ginko Biloba
    Senility and mental weakness. Cannot perform routine tasks or training
    Trembling and cramping of limbs

Lobelia Inflata
    Senile emphysema
    Initial inability to take a deep breath after rest; > walking
    General weakness leading to collapse
    Cramps in hind legs

Natrum Muriaticum
    Anaemia and emaciation
    Weakness of limbs
    Polydipsia. Much urine with low specific gravity (chronic nephritis)

References

Landsberg, G. (1998). Behavioural problems in the geriatric dog and cat. *Veterinary International* **10**(2).
Wills, J. and Wolf, A. *Handbook of Feline Medicine*. Oxford: Pergamon Press.

Chapter 30

The Homeopathic Approach to Neoplasia

General Considerations

It must always be remembered that, homeopathically, neoplasia is not a disease; it is an end product of an ongoing disease process. Since the pathology is the result of a malfunction, it follows that the pathological tendency and manifestation cannot be reversed as long as the malfunction persists. The cutting or burning-out of lesions does nothing for the underlying condition, which will in most cases return in some form. It may be considered essential, for a variety of reasons, to deal radically with a lesion, but unless the basic imbalances are addressed no complete cure will be achieved.

The practice of routinely removing what are considered as benign lumps must be viewed with caution. The phenomenon of the removal of one wart resulting in the appearance of several more is well known. In one sense this is not harmful, as the centrifugal direction of the body's reaction is maintained. But there is always the risk that unnecessary interference will finally block the direction of cure and result in a reversal of the disease process, and a driving inwards of the pathology.

While suppressive treatment of disease forms part of the aetiology of neoplasia, other factors are also involved. Suppressive treatment essentially stops the body behaving naturally, and any medication or management procedure that does not allow the body to function normally can also be regarded as a form of suppression. In addition there is the influence of carcinogenic agents, but whereas in the conventional field these are regarded as the 'cause', homeopathically they are viewed as the trigger which acts in a susceptible body. That susceptibility arises from the miasmatic make-up of the individual, which in turn exists as a result of previous exposures and procedures. These experiences are not necessarily confined to the present lifetime, and, as discussed in Chapter 11, miasmatic influences are seen clinically to be capable of passing from and to other generations.

Although initially these passages are not hereditary in the conventional sense it is possible that they can become so, and possible mechanisms whereby this can occur have been outlined (Elliott 1995; Spink 2001). While – from the homeopathic point of view – neoplasia is part of the chronic disease picture, it can on occasion quickly become life-threatening. In these cases it must be viewed as an acute flare-up of a chronic condition and treated accordingly with a suitably aggressive approach. Aggressive conventional therapy may well be suppressive in nature, and so this should be pursued homeopathically instead if possible.

The general principle of treatment on two levels is well established, with a constitutional remedy being given in moderate or high potency in conjunction with a local remedy in low potency. This principle can be applied to neoplasia but there is often one important modification. The situation will sometimes be met in cases of highly malignant tumours where the overall vital force of the patient is weakened to a degree while the energy of the local lesion is high. In these cases it may be necessary to use a local remedy in higher potency for a short time, with the deeper level of treatment being maintained at a more moderate level.

Because of the nature of the condition, considerations of the miasms must figure largely in the approach to treatment. The miasmatic balance in a particular case will vary, and this is one of the instances where histopathology can be of assistance in remedy selection. The miasms that are most prominent in neoplasia are Sycosis and Syphilis, but it must not be forgotten that all three miasmatic influences are present in all cases. In general terms, the more malignant the conventional classification, the greater the influence of Syphilis. But even in a so-called benign neoplasm, sycotic activity will be increased and the syphilitic miasm will be present to some degree. Evidence from the laboratory and radiography can assist in determining the exact balance. As in all chronic disease the totality of symptoms is the ideal basis of prescribing, but with neoplasia the presenting miasm must always be considered and addressed. As treatment progresses, a new miasmatic picture may emerge and this will influence the subsequent choice of remedy.

It must always be remembered that the neoplasm is only part of the total chronic disease picture, albeit the most dramatic. In the course of treatment other aspects of the chronic picture may appear and their significance in relation to Hering's Law, and the desirable outward movement of symptoms, is important when assessing the progress of a case.

The question of the use of miasmatic nosodes such as Carcinosin and Scirrhinum (see below) in treatment has been the subject of much controversy. One view is that, because of the advanced pathology that a neoplasm represents, the use of such remedies runs a high risk of aggravation, which is unacceptable in malignancies. A proving would of course be equally fraught with danger. The use of the LM potencies can be useful in this regard, as they can be used on a regular basis over a period of time, and one of the indications for their use is in cases where there is an advanced state of pathology. Other techniques, such as plussing, that vary the potency of each dose of the remedy can also be employed to reduce the risk of these complications. One great virtue of these remedies is that they carry within them the imprint of the miasmatic imbalance that is at the root of the condition, and hence they can be used to counteract the same imbalance when it is found in the clinical situation. The use of these and other strongly miasmatic remedies can be of great assistance in the treatment of neoplasia. Their use, alternating with more locally-acting remedies, can achieve much. These local remedies will usually have a strong organ affinity. The use of carcinogens such as Tabacum, X-ray or other agent in homeopathic potency has also been advocated (Montfort 2000).

The constitutional approach is also of great use, although some caution is necessary – the initial use of a well-selected constitutional remedy may tip the balance in the wrong direction if the patient is weak. In these cases it is usually best to begin treatment with a local or strongly miasmatic remedy and then use the constitutional remedy later.

Although resolution can be achieved in some cases, in many it is a matter of control, and in these situations the continuous use of appropriate remedies should not be rejected. Precautions as outlined above must be considered, and the alternation of remedies functioning at different levels provides a further margin of safety. But if the body needs the remedies there is no risk of any adverse effects by giving them.

Of vital importance as an adjunct to remedies is the stimulation and support of the immune system. Vitamins C and E, together with other antioxidants should be employed. Preparations based on herbs and fungi are also used to give support and stimulation to the immune system, and clinical experience indicates that they are of help. Iscador, an extract of mistletoe prepared by anthroposophical methods (which have similarities to the homeopathic process of potentisation), is often advocated in the treatment of neoplasia, and its use and results have been closely studied. Whilst undoubtedly being of assistance, its role also appears to be essentially one of supporting the immune system. As such, of course, its use is entirely compatible with homeopathy. Mistletoe is also used as a homeopathic preparation (Viscum Album), either on its own or in combination with other remedies. A 12c potency has been recorded as being the most effective (Elliott 2002).

Major Modalities and Rubrics

Rubrics such as 'cancerous affections' and those of the basic miasms must not be relied on to a great extent, as they are too general and non-specific in their range. As the best approaches involve the constitutional picture, repertorisation is based on the usual hierarchy of symptoms discussed in Chapter 6. Considerations of the location of the growth(s) can be useful, as can the consistency of any tissues involved in the neoplastic process. Pain, where it can be accurately assessed, is valuable. The rubrics will be found throughout the repertory. It cannot be stressed too much that prescribing must not become unduly biased towards the pathological aspects of the case.

Remedies of Major Use

Arsenicum Album

This is in the first rank of polychrest remedies and the widespread destructive nature of its action makes it of common use in malignancy. It has a tonic effect on all systems and can be used as a general support, irrespective of where the neoplasia is located.

The great debility coupled with burning pain and restlessness are mirrored by many advanced cases of malignancy, and its use in high potency will do much to alleviate the terminal stages of the condition. In addition to the Album, the other Arsenicum compounds must not be forgotten in this context, especially Arsenicum Iodatum. Malignancies of the endocrine glands, the lymphoid tissues, the tongue and the face may call particularly for its use.

Conium

Great hardness of tissues and especially of glands is a marked feature with this remedy. The bones are also affected with swelling of joints and weakness in the limbs. It is often indicated in the older animal. There is a tendency to ulceration.

Trauma as an aetiology is an indication for Conium, especially of the mammary glands.

Mammary tumours may show enlargement linked to the oestrus cycle. Although stabbing pains are described in relation to Conium, conditions requiring it are usually painless on palpation.

Conditions affecting glands of all kinds, the prostate, liver, testicles, lips, and stomach will often call for this remedy. Many rodent ulcers will respond.

The Miasmatic and Cancer Nosodes

Carcinosin and Scirrhinum are the two cancer nosodes of most use. Both are produced from cases of mammary neoplasia. They are hence of epithelial origin and are most indicated in tumours arising in such tissues. Carcinosin has much fear and sensitivity in its picture and the lesions are painful. There is a tendency to ulceration, which usually has a strong smell. The picture has many similarities with Argentum Nitricum.

Scirrhinum has many overlaps with Phosphorus. Animals are thin, chilly, desire cold drinks, and are fearful. It is particularly indicated in glandular affections when the glands are hard. In humans the pains are said to be more severe than with Carcinosin but this can be difficult to quantify in animals.

Syphilinum is the nosode of the syphilitic miasm. It has the syphilitic modality of < sunset to sunrise. Pain, especially of bones, and foul-smelling ulceration are features. There is enlargement of glands, and it may be of use in conditions in animals where there is the glandular swelling resembling Hodgkin's disease in humans.

Medorrhinum corresponds to the sycotic miasm. It is particularly associated with the urogenital system. There is an increase in discharges that are often green in colour. It has the general modality of < sunrise to sunset.

Tuberculinum is often required, mainly as an intercurrent remedy, in cases of neoplasia. The wasting aspects of its picture may be applicable, and in addition the syphilitic aspect of its miasmatic make-up give prescribing indications at that level.

Due to the miasmatic nature of neoplasia the psoric nosode (Psorinum) has little place in treatment.

Phosphorus

As well as being one of the leading constitutional remedies, there is a strong syphilitic influence in the remedy. This shows itself in the destructive tendency that is present in all conditions requiring the remedy, and is particularly marked in the types of neoplasia that require its use. Painful conditions of the bones point to its use in osteosarcoma. Its affinity with the eye should also be remembered, and it has indications in malignancy of the stomach where there is vomiting with blood. There is often rapid loss of condition and general weakness.

Thuja

This is one of the major sycotic remedies and its main sites of action are the skin and urogenital systems. Many warts and lipomata are helped by it, and this includes internal papillomata. Anal adenomata may respond. The warts have the characteristic cauliflower appearance and may bleed. Its role in relation to vaccination must not be forgotten when considering the aetiology of neoplasia. It is important as a constitutional remedy. It may be used as a local application in the form of the mother tincture, but this will only be truly effective if used in conjunction with a systemic constitutional approach. In addition to neoplasia in the urogenital system it may be of use with those involving the throat, pancreas and rectum.

Other Remedies to Consider

Asterias Rubens
   Ulceration of malignant tissues; especially the mammary glands
   Left-sided
   Induration of the mammary glands
   Painful conditions

Aurum and its salts
   Neoplasia of long bones and bones of face
   Depression due to pain
   Pain < night
   Enlargement of lymph glands

Hydrastis
   Thick, yellow, acrid, stringy discharges from all mucous surfaces
   Hard mammary tumours
   Vomiting of mucous discharges in cancer of the stomach

Enlargement of liver; jaundice

Scrophularia Nodosa
Enlargement of lymph glands. Hodgkin's and pseudohodgkin's disease
Affinity for mammary glands

Symphytum
Bone pain
Stimulates healing of fractures and soft tissues associated with joint injuries
Malignant growths of face

References

Blass, G. (1992) Demystifying miasms. *British Homeopathic Journal* **82**(3), Letter.

Buhler, W. and Leroi, R. (1969) Cancer as a disease of our times. *Soliale Hygiene* **19**.

Elliott, M. (2002) Homeopathy and Cancer – can it help this common problem? BAVHS Annual Conference.

Jones, E.G. (Reprinted 1993) *Cancer. Its Causes, Symptoms and Treatments*. New Delhi: B. Jain Publishers.

Montfort, H. (2000) A new homeopathic approach to neoplastic disease: from cell destruction to carcinogen-induced apoptosis. *British Homeopathic Journal* **98**, 78–83.

General Bibliography

Allen, H.C. (1931) *Keynotes with Nosodes* (8th edn). Philadelphia: Boericke & Tafel.

Allen, J.H. (1908) *The Chronic Miasms Psora and Pseudopsora*. Chicago. [Privately published]

Boericke, F.E. (1874) *Homeopathic Veterinary Practice*. Philadelphia: Hahnemann Publishing House.

Boericke, W. (1927) *Pocket Manual of Homeopathic Materia Medica* (9th edn). Philadelphia: Boericke & Runyon.

Boger, C.M. (1931) *A Synoptic Key to Materia Medica* (4th edn). Parkersburg, Virginia. [Published by the author]

Clarke, J.H. (1901, 1925) *Dictionary of Practical Materia Medica* (3 vols). London: Homoeopathic Publishing Company.

Day, C.E.I. (1990) *Homoeopathic Treatment of Small Animals*. Saffron Walden: C.W. Daniel.

Day, C.E.I. (1995) *Homoeopathic Treatment of Beef and Dairy Cattle*. Beaconsfield: Beaconsfield Publishers.

Gibson, D.M. (1987) *Studies of Homoeopathic Remedies*. Beaconsfield: Beaconsfield Publishers.

Gooch, M. (ed.) (1998, 2002) *Homeopathic thesaurus: key terms to be used in homeopathy. Homint for the European Committee for Homeopathy (ECH)*. Karlsruhe, Germany & Brussels, Belgium. www.homeopathyeurope.org

Hahnemann, C.F.S. (1896) *Chronic Diseases, Their Specific Nature and Homoeopathic Treatment* (translated by Louis H. Tafel). Philadelphia: Boericke & Tafel. [First published in 1833]

Hahnemann, C.F.S. (1852) *The Lesser Writings of Samuel Hahnemann* (translated by R.E. Dudgeon). London: Headland.

Hahnemann, C.F.S. (1880) *Materia Medicina Pura* (translated by R.E. Dudgeon). Homoeopathic Publishing Society, Liverpool. [First published in 1828.]

Hahnemann, C.F.S. (1996) *Organon of the Medical Art* (translated from *The Organon*, 6th edn, 1842 by Stephen Decker and edited by Wenda Brewster O'Reilly). Redmond: Birdcage Books.

Hunter, F.E. (2004) *Everyday Homeopathy for Animals*. Beaconsfield:

Beaconsfield Publishers.

Kent, J.T. (1932) *Lectures on Homeopathic Materia Medica* (4th edn). Philadelphia: Boericke & Tafel.

Kent, J.T. (1932) *Lectures on Homeopathic Philosophy* (2nd edn). Chicago: Ehrhart & Karl.

Koehler, G. (1986) *Handbook of Homeopathy*. Wellingborough: Thorsons.

MacLeod, G. (1983) *Veterinary Materia Medica*. Saffron Walden: C.W. Daniel.

Murphy, R. (2000) *Homeopathic Remedy Guide*. Blacksburg, Virginia: Homeopathic Academy of North America Press. [Originally issued as *The Lotus materia medica of homeopathic & spagyric medicines* (1995). Pagosa Springs, Colorado: Lotus Star Academy.]

Phatak, S.R. (1988) *Materia Medica of Homeopathic Medicines*. London: Foxlee–Vaughan Publishers.

Roberts, H.A. (1936) *Principles and Art of Cure by Homeopathy; a Modern Textbook*. London: Homoeopathic Publishing Company.

Sankaran, R. (1994) *The Substance of Homoeopathy* (2nd edn). Mumbai, India: Homoeopathic Medical Publishers.

Sankaran, R. (1999) *The Spirit of Homoeopathy* (3rd edn). Mumbai, India: Homoeopathic Medical Publishers.

Schoen, A. and Wynn, S. (1998) *Complementary and Alternative Veterinary Medicine*. London: Mosby.

Schroyens, F. (2001) *Synthesis – Repertorium Homeopathicum Syntheticum* (8.1 edn). London: Homeopathic Book Publishers.

Swayne, J. (ed.) (1998) *International Dictionary of Homeopathy*. Edinburgh: Churchill Livingstone.

Vermeulen, F. (2002) *Prisma – the Arcana of Materia Medica Illuminated*. Haarlem, The Netherlands: Emryss Publishers.

Vithoulkas, G. (1980) *The Science of Homeopathy*. New York: Grove Press.

Winston, J. (1999) *The Faces of Homeopathy*. Tawa, New Zealand: Great Auk Publishing.

Wolff, H.G. (1998) *Homeopathic Medicine For Dogs*. Saffron Walden: C. W. Daniel.

Yasgur, J. (1998) *Homeopathic Dictionary and Holistic Health Reference* (4th edn). Greenville, PA: Van Hoy Publishers.

Glossary

> Better for, ameliorated by.

< Worse for, aggrevated by.

ALLOPATHY Treatment with medicines whose effects bear no relation to the symptoms of the disease in the patient.

ANTIPATHY Treatment with medicines whose effects are the opposite to the symptoms of the disease in the patient.

CAUSALITY The attribution of an initiating cause to the disease.

CENTESIMAL SCALE The scale of dilution which employs a ratio of 1:100. Remedies prepared in this way are designated 'c', e.g. Sulphur 6c.

COMMON SYMPTOM A symptom which is common to the majority of cases of the named disease being treated. Common symptoms are of little value in prescribing, as they do not assist in individualising the patient.

COMPLEMENTARY REMEDY A homeopathic remedy whose action complements (or enhances) that of the main remedy prescribed in a case.

COMPLEX HOMEOPATHY The use of mixtures of homeopathic remedies.

CONCOMITANT SYMPTOM A symptom exhibited by the patient concurrently with the main presenting symptom.

CONSTITUTION The tendency for a patient to exhibit symptoms which correspond to a particular homeopathic medicine, no matter what the disease. The pattern is identified mainly by reference to an individual's mental and general characteristics when in health, and to their mental and general symptoms when in a state of disease.

CONSTITUTIONAL PRESCRIBING The prescription of a homeopathic medicine according to the patient's constitution.

DECIMAL SCALE The scale of potency which employs a ratio of 1:10. Remedies prepared in this way are designated 'x' or 'D', e.g. Sulphur 6x or D6.

DYNAMISATION Potentisation.

GENERAL SYMPTOM A symptom appertaining to the whole patient, such as a desire or aversion for a particular food, or seeking warmth.

HERING'S LAW The observation that cure resulting from the administration of a homeopathic remedy follows a recognised pattern.

HIERARCHY OF SYMPTOMS In the analysis of a case, the placing of symptoms in their order of importance.

HOMEOPATHY The treatment of disease with a substance which, when administered to a healthy patient, is capable of reproducing the symptom complex exhibited by the patient.

HOMEOPATHIC REMEDY A medicine prescribed on homeopathic principles; also in general usage to describe a potentised medicine.

INIMICAL REMEDY A homeopathic remedy which interferes with the action of the main remedy.

INTERCURRENT REMEDY When one homeopathic remedy is repeated, a second homeopathic remedy prescribed in between doses of the first remedy.

ISOPATHY The treatment of a disease with a potentised remedy prepared from the causative agent.

KEYNOTE SYMPTOM A symptom which is highly characteristic of a particular homeopathic remedy.

LATERALITY The propensity for the symptom picture, either of a patient or of a homeopathic remedy, to affect one side of the body.

LM POTENCY The scale of dilution in the preparation of a homeopathic remedy which uses a ratio of 1:50,000.

LOCAL SYMPTOM A symptom appertaining to a physical division of the body.

MENTAL SYMPTOM A symptom appertaining to the mental and emotional aspects of the patient.

MIASM A tendency towards expressing a consistent pattern of response to all challenges.

MODALITY Factor which changes a symptom; a general modality affects the whole individual, whereas a local modality affects a local symptom only.

MOTHER TINCTURE Alcoholic extract of plant material used as the basis for the preparation of a homeopathic remedy.

NOSODE A homeopathic remedy prepared from disease material or pathogenic organisms.

NWS 'Never Well Since.' The existence of a strong precipitating factor in the past for the chronic disease process for which the patient is presented.

PARTICULAR SYMPTOM Local symptom.

POLYCHREST A homeopathic remedy whose materia medica includes a broad range of symptoms and therefore has widespread uses.

POTENCY The healing strength of a homeopathic remedy expressed as the degree to which the source material has been diluted.

POTENTISATION The process of dilution and succussion developed by Hahnemann in the preparation of a homeopathic remedy.

PROVING The process of eliciting the symptom picture of a remedy by administering it to healthy individuals. The remedy may be in material or potentised form.

REMEDY PICTURE The sum of the symptoms associated with a particular homeopathic remedy.

REPERTORY A lexicon of symptoms which allows cross-referencing of homeopathic medicines.

SIMILIA SIMILIBUS CURENTUR 'Let likes be cured by likes.' The principle of homeopathy.

SIMILLIMUM The remedy that most closely matches the total symptoms of the patient.

SRP 'Strange, Rare and Peculiar.' A symptom which is unusual and characteristic of the patient. Of the highest order of importance in selecting the appropriate homeopathic remedy.

SUCCUSSION The process of agitating a remedy in order to potentise it, by beating the vial containing it against a solid surface.

TOTALITY The sum of a patient's symptomatology, to be used in selecting a homeopathic remedy.

TRITURATION The process of grinding an insoluble substance in lactose powder in order to render it soluble and therefore suitable for potentisation.

UNICIST PRESCRIBING The prescription of only one homeopathic remedy at a time.

VITAL FORCE The life energy of an organism, which maintains the body in harmony, and on the balance of which health depends.

Useful Addresses and Contact Points

AUSTRALIA

Australian Association of Holistic Veterinarians (AAHV).
  Tel: 08 8338 0005; Fax: 08 8338 0007;
  Email: douglaswilson@ozemail.com.au;
  www.ava.com.au/content/AAHV/index.html
Homeopathic Medical Group. Tel: 02 9416 2259;
  Email: nicamfoh@value.com.au

Pharmacies

Brauer, P.O. Box 234, 1 Para Road, Tanunda SA 5352.
  Tel: 08 8563 2932; www.brauer.com.au
Martin & Pleasance, 123, Dover Street, Richmond, Vic. 3121.
  Tel: 03 9427 7422; Email: info@mandp.com.au
Weleda Australia. Tel: 03 9723 7278

AUSTRIA

Pharmacies

Homeocur, Stadtapotheke Retz, Hauptplatz 29, 2070 Retz.
Dr Peithner GmbH, Richard Strauss Strasse 13, 1232 Wien.
  Tel: 01 616 2644; 02942 2287; www.peithner.at
Remedia GmbH, Hauptstrasse 4, 7000 Eisenstadt. Tel: 02682 62654;
  Email: hahnemann@remedia.at
Spagyra KG, Oberfeldstrasse 1a, 5082 Grodig. Tel: 06246 72370-78;
  Email: office@spagyra.at

CANADA

Canadian Professional Course in Veterinary Homeopathy,
  c/o Dr David Evans, RR3 Chester Basin, Nova Scotia, BOJ 1KO;
  Tel: 250 275 3553; Fax: 290 275 2435

Pharmacies

Boiron Canada Inc, 816 Guimond, Longueuil, Quebec.
Tel: 450 442-4000; www.boiron.com
Dolisos Canada. www.dolisos.ca
Thompson's Homeopathic Supplies, 844 Yonge Street, Toronto,
Ontario M4W 2H1. Tel: 416 922 2300;
www.thompsonshomeopathic.com

DENMARK

Foreningen for Integretet Veterinaermedicin, Postbox 429,
1505 Copenhagen V. www.net-t.dk/fiv

Pharmacies

Allergica, Funder Bygade 4, 8600 Silkeborg. Tel: 70261777
Mezina, Energivej 2, 6700 Esbjerg. Tel: 75181611
Tenna Winding Haugaard, Holmevej 13, Ledoje, 2765 Smorum.
Tel: 44654992

FINLAND

Suominen Homeopaattisen Laaketieteen Instituutti, Finnish Institute of
Homeopathic Medicine, PL 46, 00101 Helsinki.
Tel: 09 622 3090; Fax: 09 681 31470;
Email: info@ homeopatiakoulutus.fi; www.homeopatiakoulutus.fi

Pharmacy

Meilahden Apteekki, Mannerheimtie 73, 00270 Helsinki.
Tel: 09 041 0877

GERMANY

International Association for Veterinary Homeopathy,
Am Nordhang 32, 42551 Velbert. Email: office@iavh.at;
www.user.xpoint.at/iavh/default.htm

IRELAND

Pharmacies

Nelson's Homeopathic Pharmacy, 15 Duke Street, Dublin 2.
Tel: 01 679 0451
Weleda Ireland, Natural Medicine Company, Burgage, Blessington,
Co. Wicklow. Tel: 045 865575

NEW ZEALAND

Holistic Veterinary Society of the NZ Vet Association.
Tel: 04 385 7773; Fax: 04 385 7772; Email: viv.harris@clear.net.nz

Pharmacies

Lincoln Mall Pharmacy, 254 Lincoln Road, Henderson, Auckland
1208. Tel/Fax: 09 837 0905
Naturopharm, P.O. Box 952, Rotorua. Tel: 07 347 1688;
Fax: 07 347 0980; Email: info@naturo.co.nz
Selene Homeopathics, 110 Spring Street, P.O. Box 2456, Tauranga.
Tel: 07 578 3635; Fax: 07 578 3690; Email: selene.hom@xtra.co.nz
Simillimum Pharmacy, 20 Panama Street, Wellington.
Tel: 04 499 9242; www.natracare.net.nz
Weleda NZ, P.O. Box 8132, Te Mata Peak Road, Havelock North.
Tel: 06 877 7394; www.weleda.co.nz

NORWAY

Pharmacy

Apoteket Nordstjemen, Oslo & Sandefjord.

SOUTH AFRICA

Complementary Veterinary Medicine Group, c/o Dr J. Fraser,
P.O. Box 30310, Mayville 4058. Tel: 031 2614847
Dr S. Hayes, P.O. Box 269, Howard Place, 7450. Tel: 021 5310477

Pharmacies

Homeopathix Trading Co., P.O. Box 11540, Hatfield 0028.
Tel: 012 365 1224
Natura, P.O. Box 35189, Menlo Park 0102. Tel: 012 346 1771
Pharma Natura, P.O. Box 494, Bergvlei 2012. Tel: 011 445 6000
Weleda SA, P.O. Box 5502, Johannesburg 2000

SWEDEN

Drogcentralen, Bergfotsgatan 7, 43121 Molndal. Tel: 30223005

UNITED KINGDOM

Faculty of Homeopathy, 29 Park Street West, Luton LU1 3BE.
Tel: 0870 444 3955; Fax: 0870 444 3960;
Email: info@trusthomeopathy.org

British Homeopathic Association, 29 Park Street West, Luton
LU1 3BE. Tel: 0870 444 3950; Email: info@trusthomeopathy.org
British Association of Homeopathic Veterinary Surgeons, Chinham
House, Stanford in the Vale, Faringdon, Oxon SN7 8NQ.
Tel: 01367 718115; www.bahvs.com
British Homeopathic Library, Glasgow Homeopathic Hospital,
1053 Great Western Road, Glasgow G12 0XQ. Tel: 0141 211 1617;
Fax: 0141 211 1610; Email: hominform@dial.pipex.com

Pharmacies

Ainsworths Homeopathic Pharmacy, 36 New Cavendish Street,
London W1G 8UF. Tel: 020 7935 5330; Fax: 020 7486 4313;
www.ainsworth.com
Buxton & Grant, 176 Whiteladies Road, Bristol BS8 2XU.
Tel: 0117 973 5025
Freeman's Homeopathic Pharmacy, 20 Main Street, Busby, Glasgow
G76 8DU. Tel: 0141 644 1165; Fax: 0141 644 5735;
Email: orders@freechem.co.uk; www.freemans.uk.com
Galen Homeopathics, Lewell Mill, West Stafford, Dorchester, Dorset
DT2 8AN. Tel: 01305 263996; Fax: 01305 250792
E. Gould & Son, 14 Crowndale Road, London NW1 1TT.
Tel: 020 7387 1888; www.alternativepharmacy.co.uk
Helios Homeopathic Pharmacy, 89-97 Camden Road, Tunbridge
Wells, Kent TN1 2QR. Tel: 01892 537254; Fax: 01892 546850;
Email: pharmacy@helios.co.uk; www.helios.co.uk
Nelsons Homoeopathic Pharmacy, 73 Duke Street, London W1K 5BY.
Tel: 020 76293118; www.nelsonshomoeopathy.co.uk
Weleda UK Ltd, Heanor Road, Ilkeston DE7 8DR. Tel: 0115 944 200;
Fax: 0115 944 210; www.weleda.co.uk

USA

American Holistic Veterinary Medical Association,
2214 Old Emmorton Road, Bel Air, MD 21015. Tel: 410 569 0795;
Fax: 410 569 2346
Academy of Veterinary Homeopathy, P.O. Box 9280, Wilmington,
DE 19809. Tel/Fax: 866 652 1590; www.theavh.org
Professional Course in Veterinary Homeopathy, Animal Natural
Health Centre, 1238 Lincoln, Eugene, OR 97401.
Tel: 541 342 7665; Email: office@drpitcairn.com;
www.drpitcairn.com

Pharmacies

Acres USA, 5321 Industrial Oaks Boulevard, Ste 128, Houston, TX 78735. Tel: 512 892 4400

Boiron USA, Box 449, 6 Campus Boulevard, Bldg A, Newtown Square, PA 19073. Tel: 0800-BLU-TUBE; www.boiron.com

Dolisos USA, 3014 Rigel Avenue, Las Vegas, NV 89102. Tel: 0800 365 4767; www.dolisosamerica.com

Heel Inc., 116090 Cochiti SE, Albuquerque, NM 87123. Tel: 0800 621 7644; www.heelusa.com

Homeopathic Educational Services, 2124 Kittredge Street, Berkeley, CA 94704. Tel: 510 649 0294; www.homeopathic.com

Nature's Way, 10 Mountain Springs Parkway, Springville, UT 84663. Tel: 0800 876 9505; www.naturesway.com

Standard Homeopathic, P.O. Box 61067, 210 West 131st Street, Los Angeles, CA 90061. Tel: 0800 624 9659; www.hylands.com

Washington Homeopathic Pharmacy, 33 Fairfax Street, Berkeley Springs, WV 25411. Tel: 304 258 2541; www.homeopathyworks.com

Weleda USA, 175 North Route 9VV, Congers, NY 10920. Tel: 0800 241 1030; www.weleda.com

Index

abdominal pain 208, 209
abortion 225
Academy of Veterinary Homeopathy 12
ACE inhibitors 249–50
Aconitum Napellus (Aconite) 17, 187, 198, 276
Actea Spicata 238
ACTH 259
acupuncture 182, 244
acute disease 36-7, 48–9
  case-taking 62
  conversion to chronic 52–3
  herd/flock/kennel/cattery situation 65–6
  prescribing 87–8, 89, 102–3
  response to treatment 93–4
Addison's disease 259
administration (of remedies) 38–40
  frequency 89, 90
  routes 38–9, 91
Adonis Vernalis 253
ageing 278–80
aggravation 46-7, 99–101
  antidoting 101
  externalising 100–1
  therapeutic 94, 99–100
aggression 272, 275, 276
Agnus Castus 234
Allen, H.C. 73
Allen, J.H. 55
allergodes 139
allergy 140, 262–3
Allium Cepa 193
allopathy 1–2, 294
Ammonium Carbonicum 203, 251
anal glands 121
anger 273
angina pectoris 252
Anthracinum 139
anthrax 10, 139
anthropomorphism 66
anti-inflammatory agents 44, 52, 119, 261

see also corticosteroids; non-steroidal anti-inflammatory drugs
antibiotics 44, 52, 119, 182, 261
antibodies
  maternal 167, 168
  response to vaccination 164–6, 171, 174
antidoting of remedies 101
antifungal agents 261
antigen 165
Antimonium Tartaricum 203
antipathy 1–2, 294
anxiety 273, 274
Apis Mellifica 28, 187–8, 242, 243
appetite 112, 113, 114, 115
Argentum Nitricum 198, 274
Aristolochia Clematitis 259
Arndt-Schultz law 16-17
Arnica Montana
  indications 188, 241, 281
  prescribing 84, 89
  research 16
Arsenicum Album
  constitutional type 109–10
  indications 195–6, 201, 207–8, 213, 219, 266-7, 284, 288
  repertorisation 78, 80–1
  research studies 16, 21
arthritis 67–8, 83, 118, 236, 239–40
ascites 212, 213
aspergillosis 193
aspirin 236
Asterias Rubens 290
asthma 56, 199
atopic dermatitis 78, 80–1
atopy 85, 120, 261–2, 264
audit, clinical 22
Aurum and its salts 290
Aurum Metallicum 136
autoimmune diseases 42, 170
autonosode 139, 140
Avogadro's number 14, 32–3

302

Index

osteochondritis dissecans (OCD) 236, 237
osteosarcoma 290
outbreaks, disease 141
ovarian problems 258
owners
    administration of remedy 94–5
    case-taking *see* case-taking
oxygenoid type 124

pain
    injury-related 188, 189, 190
    musculoskeletal problems 237, 238–9
palliation 98–9
Paracelsus 2
paralysis 85, 242, 246, 283
parasites 206, 263
particular symptoms 5, 59, 296
parturition 20, 226, 227
Pasteur, Louis 72, 125
Paterson, John and Elizabeth 147, 149, 151, 155
pathodes 138, 172–3
pathogenetic trial, homeopathic *see* proving
pathological prescribing 84
People's Dispensary for Sick Animals 10–11
periodontal disease 116, 117
periosteal injuries 190, 191
phagocytosis 50, 129–30
Phosphorus
    constitutional type 112–13
    indications 198, 201–2, 209, 213, 219–20, 290
    laterality and 59
    miasmic conditions 136
    research studies 16, 19, 20
    selection 85
photophobia 195, 197
Phytolacca 20, 136, 229
pillules 38
Pitcairn, Richard 12
pituitary-adrenal-gonad triad 223, 229, 255–6
placebo effect 17, 23
Plumbum Metallicum 16, 246–7
plussing 34, 287
pneumonia 201–2, 203
polychrests 36, 79, 184, 296
polyuria 219
potency 29–31, 296

centesimal (c) 5, 29, 30, 93
decimal (D or x) 29, 30, 93
LM (Q) 30–1, 89–90, 93, 295
mother 31
selection 89, 91–3
potency chord 92
potentisation 5, 29–34, 296
mixtures 103
powders 38
pregnancy 226, 227
false 225, 228, 229
prescribing 87–103
constitutional *see* constitutional prescribing
dosage aspects 88–91
getting started 180
levels 83–4
methods 83–6
potency considerations 91–3
recognising the problem 87–8
Unicist 102–3, 296
see also remedies
prescription, second 101–2
primary action 46-7
Primary Certificate in Veterinary Homeopathy 12
prophylaxis, nosodes for 140–1, 173–4
prostaglandins 51, 224
prostate
cancer 232, 234
enlargement 233, 234
prostatitis 233, 234
Proteus Bach 150, 156, 159
proving 4–5, 34–5, 296
clinical 97–8, 101
pruritus (itching) 78, 80–1, 265, 266, 267, 268
psora 54, 124, 125–6, 128
bowel nosodes 152
current concepts 129, 130
recognising 133–4
remedies 136
Psorinum 138, 143
Psycho-Neuro-Endocrine-Immune (PNEI) axis 42–3
pulmonary oedema 203, 251
Pulsatilla Nigricans 86
constitutional type 113–14
indications 196, 221, 228, 233, 238–9, 267–8
pyometra 58, 227, 228
pyrexia *see* fever